Leadership training
in mental health

EDITED BY

George W. Magner AND
Thomas L. Briggs

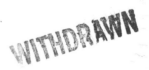

National Association of Social Workers, Inc.
2 Park Avenue, New York, New York 10016

*Grateful acknowledgment is made to the National Insti-
tute of Mental Health for a grant that made possible the
publication of this volume.*

Leadership Training
in Mental Health

Contents

Preface

The opportunity to participate in an active and exciting project such as the Leadership Training Program of the National Association of Social Workers is enhanced by the opportunity to share with a wider audience some of the components and results of the project. The several papers that comprise this volume were selected both to provide the reader with information about and an analysis of one continuing education program and to illustrate the nature of the material introduced during the program. The first and the last papers (by Magner and Cohen) deal rather specifically with the goals, process, and impact of the Leadership Training Program. The intervening papers present, in order, a conceptual framework for relating service organizations to primary community groups (Litwak) and the implementation and hazards of major program innovations (Beck and Studt).

The editors are grateful to the authors for preparation of the papers contained in this volume and their permission to include them. Special thanks go to the program participants, leaders, and advisory groups, who combined as one membership body to produce a highly successful training experience.

—G.W.M.
T.L.B.

Evolution of the leadership training program

George W. Magner

There can be no denial of the changes under way in the provision of mental health services in the United States. Beginning slowly and cautiously in the mid-1950s and rapidly accelerating in the 1960s, the demands for change were perhaps best symbolized by the unprecedented 1963 message to Congress of the late President John F. Kennedy. In calling for "a bold new approach" he signaled the beginning of a period in which a developing federal social policy would have an impact on mental health services throughout the nation. The earlier report by the Joint Commission on Mental Health and Illness had preceded this presidential action and frankly and clearly set forth the deficiencies in programs and manpower.[1]

---

[1] *Action for Mental Health,* Final Project of the Joint Commission on Mental Illness and Health (New York: Basic Books, 1961).

Emphasis on these two actions does not deny the influence and importance of earlier developments such as the use since the 1950s of a range of psychopharmaceuticals, experimentation with "open" hospitals, stress on the therapeutic milieu, and other innovations. However, the significance of the commission's report, the President's message, and the later congressional action lies in the potential of federal policy and legislation to effect change on a nationwide basis. While the federal government, largely through the National Institute of Mental Health, had been supporting research and training activities for a number of years, the time had yet to come when such support would encompass broad programs of service.

The first federal programs of this nature were established in 1961 by the development of the Hospital Improvement Program. This legislation authorized expenditure of federal funds on a nonmatching basis for the improvement of clinical services in state hospitals and state institutions for the mentally retarded. Such legislation suggests recognition of the reality of the situation: that despite the promise of alternatives to institutionalization, the majority of seriously ill mental patients were still being cared for in large, often isolated, and generally poorly staffed state hospitals and schools. Emphasis of the Hospital Improvement Program was therefore on the improvement of treatment within these institutions. Related legislation enacted the following year made funds available to these same institutions for expanded programs of in-service staff training essential to the aim of improved care.

In rapid succession two major legislative enactments placed federal resources squarely behind the comprehensive community mental health approach as a singular model for coping with the nation's mental health needs. PL 88-164 (construction) and PL 89-105 (staffing) provided federal funds, on a declining basis (75–30 percent over fifty-two months), to local health organizations, public or private, that conformed to federal guidelines for the provision of service. Such availability of federal moneys has served as an impetus to local development, with a consequent manifold increase in the number of community mental health centers.

It is not the intent of this paper to provide an analysis or critique of federal legislation or the community mental health center model. However, an awareness of such developments—of the fluid nature of service delivery—is essential to an understanding of the rationale for continuing professional education such as that provided by the Leadership Training Program of the National Association of Social Workers.

Implications of New Developments

The social worker (and many other professionals) in mental health had been immersed for a number of years in a narrow and limited service system. With the exception of the few persons engaged in private practice, social workers were employed in one of the two dominant mental health institutions: the state hospital or school for the retarded and the so-called community clinic. The former was likely to be a custodial institution, long isolated and insulated from political and public scrutiny, while the latter more closely resembled a semiprivate practice, with formidable administrative barriers to service. Community service by the state hospital or state school was mainly limited to confinement of those members the community considered sufficiently deviant for exclusion. Similar limitations were apparent in service provided by community clinics, which operated on a rigid patient-therapist model, with admission to service reserved for the select few who met the criteria imposed by the elite triad of mental health professionals—the psychiatrist, psychologist, and social worker. Admission standards often served the interests of the therapist rather than the community. From a systems view both the institution and the clinic were largely closed and isolated from their environment.[2]

The shift to a comprehensive community mental health approach has had enormous implications for professional practice and the mental health practitioner. Without elaboration, the following comprise the major ones:

1. The comprehensive approach not only suggests an array of available therapeutic agents, but further suggests that the facilities be available and accessible to all segments of the population. This

---

[2] For an exposition of mental health procedures that foster this type of isolation, *see* Elaine Cumming, *Systems of Social Regulation* (New York: Atherton Press, 1968), pp. 74–75.

dictum was never before observed and has necessitated not only changes in service delivery patterns but critical analysis of therapeutic techniques.

2. The manpower crisis has been made more acute. The combination of personnel shortages and recognition that the classically trained professional might be less effective than others in fulfilling certain tasks has led to extensive modification of thinking about manpower utilization. Wide use of indigenous workers and the mushrooming of training programs for a variety of mental health technicians have caused the professional role to be examined carefully. There is an explicit assumption that the mental health professional will move into a broader leadership and training role as more direct service tasks are undertaken by others.

3. Meaningful involvement by community representatives, including some recipients of proposed services, is expected on a scale rarely encountered in the earlier protected and limited mental health programs. The old cliché, "mental health is everyone's business," was believed by few professionals, and true consumer participation greatly disturbed the notion that essential services could and should be provided only by those few trained to do so.

4. The requirement that federal funding be supplemented by state and local moneys has led to a much more intensive political monitoring of mental health programs. As the use of public tax money has increased, so has the interest of public officials. The mental health professional who had long maintained an air of aloofness from political considerations suddenly discovered that program survival might depend on his ability to negotiate successfully with these forces—and few were prepared by training and disposition to do this.

The several implications noted do not represent an exhaustive list. They will, however, serve to illustrate the dilemma in which many mental health professionals found themselves—given for the first time an opportunity to provide something more than a token community service, they were less than convinced of either their enthusiasm or their ability to do so. This, then, was the general position of social work in mental health as perceived by the formulators of the NASW Leadership Training Program.

NASW Leadership Training Program

In 1963 NASW had begun, with the aid of an NIMH grant, a three-year staff development program conducted along traditional lines and aimed at enhancing the training capacity of supervisory personnel in public and private mental institutions and schools for the retarded. The mechanism—the Hospital Supervisors' Institute—was viewed as one that would ultimately improve the institutional service provided to patients and their families. Although it was not planned to do so, it coincided with the development of the Hospital Improvement Program of NIMH, the first of the major federal service-oriented programs and one that provided nonmatching grants for projects designed to improve institutional services.

By the third and final year of the Hospital Supervisors' Institute program it became apparent that, while the individual institutes had been well received and had involved representatives from most institutions in the geographic areas served, emphasis on the usual staff development methods and techniques was simply insufficient.[3] By this time (1965) the pressure toward change had begun to build and the demand was for programs that would serve in a meaningful fashion those population segments that had remained all but ignored.

The Hospital Supervisors' Institutes did not view change as a central objective. In retrospect institutions for the mentally ill and retarded were accepted as the predominant service institutions and there was relatively little impetus to substitute radically different models. True, the deficiencies were identified and explicated. However, emphasis was placed on a staff development process that would make the institutions more functional and not on any type of systemic change. With recognition that this was not enough, a modified proposal emerged that was later to be called the Leadership Training Program. Funded in 1965 by NIMH, the

---

[3] With the exception of one year when several far western states were included in an extra institute, the two geographic areas served were the Southeast (eleven states) and the Southwest (eight states). Of the eligible institutions in these areas, about 80 percent were represented at one or more of the institutes during the three-year program.

Leadership Training Program completed its first three-year cycle in June 1968 and is now in its second cycle.

Purpose and Goals

The purpose and goals differed philosophically from those of the Hospital Supervisors' Institute. The pace of change, greatly accelerated by the federal legislation mentioned earlier, demanded leadership by mental health professionals who were sophisticated not only as clinicians but as managers, negotiators, and program analysts. Sensitivity to ethnic, class, and social differences was as essential as responsiveness to political mandates and public social policy. Specifically, the major goals of the program were as follows:

1. To examine the position of mental health within the broader social welfare system and its interdependence with other fields.

2. To achieve a greater understanding of the organizational structures by which mental health services are now delivered and to review alternate models.

3. To heighten the understanding of the interaction between and the mutual dependency of the formal mental health organization and the array of significant community forces.

4. To increase awareness on the part of social workers of the public social policy issues that increasingly bear on mental health services (legislation and legislative processes, governmental programs, financial considerations, and so on).

5. To understand more clearly certain essential components of administrative and leadership behavior (negotiation processes, necessary alignments, sources and uses of power, the element of personal risk, and the like).

At the risk of using what sometimes seems to be an overworked word, perhaps the simplest way to describe the basic aim of the program is the attainment of power. The basic premise suggests that the social work professional should play an expanded role in the delivery of mental health services. Power, then, is meant in the sense in which Lasswell and Kaplan used it—as "participation in the making of decisions"—or in the meaning of Etzioni—as a meaningful share of available resources.[4]

Social workers in the mental health field have an increasing amount of *ascribed* power—power that is given as a result of professional roles, training, and accepted competence. This power base, however, remains limited and much of social work influence and participation in decision-making must be *achieved*. In a paper given at one of the leadership training sessions, Wax noted the strain of such achievement: "Power does not come to the passive, the timid, the indolent, the defeated or the obsequious. The development and exercise of power is a strenuous business, requiring energy, conviction, courage, resilience, and cool pragmatism."[5]

It should perhaps be added that power is not sought for its own sake. There is an obvious assumption underlying the program: that the knowledge base, the organizational capability, and the value system of social work place this professional group in a position to affect positively the delivery of mental health services. Given this assumption, the task is how best to ensure that social work will participate in the most meaningful fashion.

In contrast to the earlier Hospital Supervisors' Institutes, which sought to improve institutional services, the Leadership Training Program gave emphasis to the identification and selection of those individual social workers, regardless of agency affiliation, who were in or moving toward positions of leadership in the mental health field—individual social workers who had demonstrated interest in departing from the traditional patterns of practice and the ability to do so. Once this was done, the task of the training program was seen as twofold: (1) to add sufficiently to the conceptual and knowledge base of the participants so as to enhance their effectiveness as leaders and (2) to achieve an attitudinal shift by which the participant would begin to view himself in a leadership role.

---

[4] Harold D. Lasswell and Abraham Kaplan, *Power and Society* (New Haven: Yale University Press, 1965), p. 75; Amitai Etzioni, *The Active Society* (New York: Fress Press, 1968), chap. 13.

[5] John Wax, "Relevant Power," p. 3. Unpublished paper delivered at the NASW Leadership Training Institute, Chicago, April 1967.

The first of these tasks has been viewed as crucial. Part of leadership involves risk-taking, and risk can be minimized by competence and knowledge. If the individual is to seek power within an institution, the degree to which this is attained will be increased in proportion to an increase in his knowledge of the institutional norms and values, his ability to analyze the institution's structure and resources, and his capacity to negotiate with other blocs within the institution. Attitudinal change is less precise and therefore less easy to detail. However, the opportunity for interaction with those pursuing similar goals and for participation in serious decision-making can and often does produce an expanded professional set and identity. Combination of the two tasks appears essential. Leadership behavior without the requisite knowledge will be futile, as will a body of knowledge without the motivation and courage to behave as required.

Process and Methodology

Given these essentials of philosophy and objectives, it might be of value to sketch briefly the process and methodology of the Leadership Training Program. Invitations to apply to the program are issued to persons nominated by several national groups, among them the Conference of Chief Social Workers in State and Territorial Mental Health Programs, deans of schools of social work, regional and national NIMH staff members, and NASW chapter presidents. All participants are selected by a special review committee. The response to the first program was excellent: Thirteen hundred invitations were mailed, with more than 300 applications received. From this group 101 persons were selected for participation in seven workshops. These were fairly young (most falling in the 25–40 range), largely male (75 percent), and nearly all in supervisory or executive positions. All members of the program—participants, workshop leaders, and advisory committee members—were asked to make a full commitment to it. The strength of this commitment becomes apparent on examination of the attendance figures: the attrition rate for the three-year period was only 5 percent for participants; not a single workshop leader had to be replaced.

In the second program, now under way, about 200 applications were received from the 800 persons invited. An eighth workshop was added and 117 persons were selected. Again the group is largely male (80 percent), young, and in positions of responsibility. With some expansion of the definition of mental health, representatives were included from agencies not clearly identified with the field, such as antipoverty organizations and school systems, although these are in the minority.

The educational design has remained basically the same in the current as in the first program. There are two major components: annual concentrated one-week sessions and the interim periods. The concentrated sessions, or institutes, include general sessions at which major papers are presented, small workshop groups (maintained intact over the three-year period) provision of reading materials, optional site visits and films, consultation, and various informal activities. During each interim period reading lists are provided and a major written project assigned. During the first program the interim projects were all undertaken on an individual basis: some group projects are currently in progress. Also during the first program there was an attempt to provide interim consultation by the appointment of "preceptors." For several reasons this proved valuable in only a few instances and it has not been continued.

Progress during the first program involved movement from a relatively passive "student" role to active participation in the planning and programming of future sessions. The same is currently true, except that the pace of involvement has been greatly accelerated. Such acceleration reflects both the action orientation of 1969 and the presence during the first week-long session of several readymade issues: concern over scheduling a national meeting in Chicago (as a reaction to the events surrounding the Democratic National Convention), the limited number of minority group participants, and the extent of consumer participation. It suggests also that the social worker in the mental health field is undergoing a shift in role identity and that his perception of the responsibilities of leadership includes active and aggressive participation in the planning and administration of the programs with which he is affiliated.

Evaluation of the Program

While in-depth analysis of the program and its impact was not attempted, a twofold assessment was made: (1) evaluation by the participants of various program components and (2) some review of participants' career changes during the three-year period of the first program. The low attrition rate over the first three-year period suggests in itself a substantial level of satisfaction and continuing commitment on the part of the participants. This appears to be confirmed by participant rating of the program on a scale ranging from 1 ("very negative—of little or no value") through 9 ("very positive—of much value"). Results are given in Table 1.

Table 1. Participant Rating of Overall Program ($N=72$)

Rating	Number
9	31
8	20
7	13
6	4
5	4
4	0
3	0
2	0
1	0

A detailed analysis of evaluative comments made will not be presented here, but some highlights are as follows:

1. While there was a wide range of responses to individual didactic presentations, those that provided most stimulus for discussion and professional change combined two major ingredients: (a) The content had a clear theoretical base but spoke directly to questions and problems of administrative practice. (b) Presentation was made by persons who themselves represented strong social work leadership.

2. The workshop groups brought clearly into focus the issue of content versus process—an issue that is still not fully resolved. The group leader emerges as a key figure. There was some nega-

tive reaction to being "taught" or "lectured to" in the small groups, but a similar reaction when group process assumed too great a predominance over content. An ideal model might perhaps combine the two elements—providing sufficient structure to ensure discussion of relevant content but with enough flexibility and openness to allow the necessary involvement and interaction.

3. Participant reaction to such features as a small "library" and site visits was varied. If optional, they apparently are of interest and value to some, while of little value to others.

4. The interim assignments do provide an essential continuity and allow the individual to apply conceptual material within the context of his own institution. The evaluative comments reflect this but also indicate the need for more thought about the use and distribution of completed papers. There must also be an institutional response in the form of a critique or review of completed assignments. In a few instances there was a highly negative reaction when such was not forthcoming.

The second facet of the assessment—career changes—was carried out by an analysis of career movement during the period members were enrolled in the program. The data are not striking (see Table 2), but a few results will be discussed.

Table 2. Job Categories of Participants at Beginning and End of the Leadership Training Program ($N=72$)

	Number of Participants	
Job Categories	Beginning of program	Termination of program
Executive-managerial	42	45
Direct clinical practice	10	4
Social work supervision	7	3
Program consultation	6	5
University teaching–staff development [a]	4	11
Community organization–planning	3	3
Student (doctoral)	0	1

[a] Staff development is differentiated from supervision in the breakdown of job categories as having broad program responsibility such as in the position of institutional or state director of staff development.

In view of the aims of the Leadership Training Program, it is not surprising that the majority of participants occupied executive or managerial positions, and this number increased slightly over the program period. The most substantial upward change was in the university teaching–staff development category, with the number of persons almost tripling. The major decrease is seen in the two categories where social workers in mental health have traditionally been employed, direct clinical practice and supervision. At the beginning of the program these two categories encompassed 24 percent of the respondents, which was reduced to 10 percent by the end of the program.

Not shown in Table 2 is the overall job mobility. Of the 72 respondents, 27 (37 percent) changed positions during the program period, with 6 of these changes representing assumption of greater responsibility within the same organization.

Although incomplete, some data are available on the extent of NASW and other professional and civic activities. The range of NASW involvement is wide and includes 4 delegates to the 1967 Delegate Assembly, 5 chapter presidents, 7 other chapter officers, 4 chapter committee chairmen, 5 speakers at the Second NASW Professional Symposium held in San Francisco in 1968, and 3 members of national units. Thirty-six persons (50 percent) listed some NASW activity, with the political or legislative sphere mentioned with greatest frequency. One person had been elected NASW chapter "Social Worker of the Year." Forty-two persons (58 percent) were active in other civic and professional spheres—local health and welfare organizations, governors' committees, state or other policy-making bodies. Several were directly involved in political campaigns or with legislative leaders.

While a number of respondents noted that the Leadership Training Program was responsible, in part at least, for position reappraisal and change and for an increase in other professional activities, it is not possible in this type of assessment to establish a firm relationship. A review of the total activities of the respondents does suggest a deep professional commitment and involvement.

At least one concrete accomplishment resulted from the program. In a general session at the close of the second year of the first program, the group deplored the lack of an NASW position statement on community mental health. A seven-member committee (one person from each workshop group) was elected and charged with the development of such a statement. Working during and between sessions, the committee developed a position paper for ratification by the total group. This paper was subsequently approved by the Council on Social Work in Mental Health and Psychiatric Services and in March 1969 was approved by the NASW Board of Directors as the association's official position statement on community mental health.

Conclusions

The model described is but one of the possibilities for continuing professional education during a time of rather drastic change. The professional, regardless of his field, cannot quickly abandon traditional methods of functioning and thinking. It is in the nature of professional training that certain patterns of behavior—certain bases of knowledge and theory—are adopted and put to use for the general good. It would be most unfortunate—and a great public disservice—for the professional to change with each changing conception of practice.

Nonetheless change is necessary and there must be experimentation with the means by which such change can be accomplished. The Leadership Training Program is one such means. Sponsored by the professional membership association, it remains relatively flexible and need not assume the secondary position to which a school, concerned first with basic curriculum changes, might assign it. Such a model also relates directly to the field of practice, allowing a mutual influence in terms of content and process. Finally, the time and cost are not prohibitive, while the three-year period provides a continuity and a sequential series of learning experiences that go beyond the one-shot workshop or institute. The Leadership Training Program is, in essence, an exciting venture in the provision by the professional association of an ongoing educational experience for its members.

Toward a balance theory
of grass-roots community organization

Eugene Litwak

This paper represents an attempt to outline a theory of relationships between professionals and community primary groups and
to indicate how this might be used to guide social work practice.
It is an attempt to formulate a theory of grass-roots community
organization whereby "grass roots" means the relationship between
the professional and the family, neighbors, and friends of the client.
This is far from a complete analysis of community problems faced
by professionals. For instance, the relationships among bureaucratic organizations will not be discussed. Three bodies of litera-

This paper is a slightly modified version of a series of papers prepared by
Henry J. Meyer and Eugene Litwak. It is therefore only in the technical
sense of having prepared this specific version that Eugene Litwak is the
sole author. However, since there are some differences from prior works,
he assumes all responsibility.

ture will be analyzed: that seeking to highlight what the primary group (family, neighbors, friends) and the bureaucratic organization can best do, that attempting to develop the properties of the linkage mechanisms that connect them, and the theory of organizational structures that limits the kinds of linkages that can operate in a given agency.

Philosophies of Community Relations

There are at least three distinctive philosophies of how social workers should relate to the community: the separatist, the integrationist, and the balance theory. Each will be discussed in turn.

Separatist Approach

The separatist approach argues that the social worker will best operate as a professional in the confines of his office. This philosophy has several theoretical bases. First, the adoption of a Freudian or neo-Freudian theory of treatment as the major facet of social work practice suggests that treatment of the intrapsychic needs of the individual is the social worker's key job and that all pertinent information and tools for treatment can be found in the social worker–client dyad. There is no need to confront family, friends, or neighbors directly. Moreover, treatment is only successful when the client has sufficient grasp of his problem to know he needs treatment, as manifested by the fact that he has come to the social agency seeking it. As a consequence, reaching-out services to the community are neither necessary nor desirable. Finally, performing therapy is a highly developed skill requiring extensive professional training. Most important in this regard is the need for the social worker to maintain objectivity in a situation of close interpersonal involvement; therefore volunteers and amateurs must be prohibited from using such treatment procedures, since they are quite likely to introduce the personalistic demands of the primary group into the therapeutic situation. It is important that such volunteers be kept as distant from the worker as possible.

These reasons for maintaining a distance from the community are further supported by developments in sociological theory, which suggest that under the impact of modern industrialization the community primary groups such as the family are weakened, if not destroyed. Thus some speak about the loss of the family's functions in modern society.[1] Others point out that the bureaucratic organization is the best means of solving problems in an industrial society.[2] Moreover, even in those instances when the family still retains its ability to solve problems, it is unlikely to survive because of the demands of a bureaucratic organization for impersonal, transitory, specialized, or segmental relations.[3] As a consequence of all this, there seemed to be a good basis for arguing that social workers as professionals have no valid reason for heavy involvement in the local community.

The only problem with this approach is that social work professionals have found it increasingly necessary to include community primary groups in the treatment unit if they are to achieve effective results. Thus programs on delinquency have pointed out the need to treat the entire gang rather than individual members and to do so in the neighborhood milieu. This has led to the development of the youth gang worker.[4] Others have pointed out that it is necessary to treat the entire family if a given member is to be reached.[5] Still others have suggested that to cure a mental patient

---

[1] William F. Ogburn, "The Changing Functions of the Family," in Robert F. Winch and Robert McGinnis, eds., *Selected Readings in Marriage and the Family* (New York: Holt, Rinehart & Winston, 1953), pp. 74–76.

[2] H. H. Gerth and C. Wright Mills, eds., *From Max Weber: Essays in Sociology* (New York: Oxford University Press, 1964), pp. 196–224.

[3] See Joseph A. Schumpeter, *Capitalism, Socialism, and Democracy* (2d ed.; New York: Harper & Row, 1947), p. 157; Louis Wirth, "Urbanism as a Way of Life," in Paul K. Hiatt and Albert J. Reiss, Jr., eds., *Cities and Society: The Revised Reader in Urban Sociology* (New York: Free Press of Glencoe, 1957), pp. 593–594; Ferdinand Tonnies, *Fundamental Concepts of Sociology* (New York: American Book Co., 1940), pp. 18–28.

[4] See P. L. Crawford, D. I. Malamud, and James R. Dumpson, *Working with Teenage Gangs* (New York: Welfare Council of New York City, 1950).

[5] See Nathan W. Ackerman, Frances L. Beatman, and Sanford N. Sherman, eds., *Exploring the Base for Family Therapy* (New York: Family Service Association of America, 1961).

in a hospital, one must understand the community from which he came and to which he will return.[6] This has led to programs that seek to work with the family and friends of returning patients.[7] Much of this recognition that the client's primary groups must be included if the treatment process is to be successful has culminated in the concept of community mental health. In other words, there seem to be important empirical exceptions taken to a separatist point of view, exceptions that have a solid theoretical base.

Integrationist Philosophy

A second point of view currently being advocated is the opposite of the separatist philosophy and has been termed the integrationist point of view. One major group advocating this philosophy has argued that the major social problems occur among the poor and suggests that the key elements in social problems are environmental rather than intrapsychic.[8] Since the environment of the poor is considered the key variable in social work practice, the social worker must work in the community if he is to do some good. The client often has a better knowledge of his milieu and is in a better position than the social worker to make quick and flexible decisions with regard to his environment. These facts are behind the demands that indigenous leaders be put on the boards of directors of antipoverty programs and that indigenous persons rather than professionals be hired as project workers. This philosophy tends to suggest an almost complete merger of professionals and community residents.

The merger of social workers and the indigenous community primary group does not take into account the separatist objection that the professional and community member operate on the basis

---

[6] Ozzie G. Simmons and Howard E. Freeman, "Family Expectations and Post-hospital Performance of Mental Patients," *Human Relations*, Vol. 12, No. 2 (August 1959), pp. 233–242.

[7] *See* Howard E. Freeman and Ozzie G. Simmons, *The Mental Patient Comes Home* (New York: John Wiley & Sons, 1963), pp. ix–x.

[8] Richard A. Cloward and Irwin Epstein, "Private Social Welfare's Disengagement from the Poor: The Case of Family Adjustment Agencies," in Mayer N. Zald, ed., *Social Welfare Institutions* (New York: John Wiley & Sons, 1965), pp. 623–644.

of different criteria. The power of the indigenous leader is based
on trust and loyalty. All things being equal, he is likely to make
decisions that will benefit family and friends first, while the needs
of the larger community are secondary. The costs of this particularistic orientation can be seen in several related developments. The
inability of auditors of some programs dominated by indigenous
leaders to account in any "legal" manner for the way government
funds were spent often represents nepotism encouraged by primary
group ties. In part accusations of fraud are malicious attempts to
discredit a program. However, from a theoretical perspective, programs that turn funds over to indigenous leaders without special
safeguards will be vulnerable to such charges because the power
of the indigenous leader comes from his stress on nepotistic primary group ties as ideal states.

The dangers of too much closeness between professional and
primary group member can be seen from another perspective.
Professionals who work closely with indigenous groups and who
become too identified with the people with whom they are working lose sight of the larger organizational goals and eventually
have to be dropped from the agency. This is because the organization must deal with the total community and a particularistic
stress on one neighborhood might lead to discrimination against
others. The professional must always represent this point of view
to the specific neighborhood within which he is working in order
to justify why it is that the organization cannot utilize all of its
resources in that one neighborhood. When because of overidentification the professional can no longer make this distinction, he
becomes a liability to the agency. Thus problems of nepotism,
favoritism, corruption, and professional overidentification are all
manifestations of the excessive closeness of professionals and indigenous leaders.

To point out that there are some problems with the integrationist
point of view is not to question its major assumptions, such as that
environmental factors play a major role in explaining the problems
of the poor and that the professional must as a consequence work
much more closely with the poor in their communities. What it
does suggest is the need for the integrationist to make explicit how
the universalistic criteria of the professional can be kept separate

from the particularistic ones of the indigenous leader—assuming that both are needed.

The Balance Theory

As was pointed out, there are some problems in bringing indigenous persons into an organization that suggest a complete merger is not the ideal, even in the field of community organization. On the other side of the coin, trends suggest that even intrapsychic problems require close work with the total primary group or community. What is most important is the implicit assertion of a partnership arrangement. This formulation is close to that which has been called the "balance theory" of co-ordination. It states that both bureaucratic organizations (including their professionals) and community primary groups are essential elements in accomplishing most tasks and that keeping them too far apart will make the job more difficult. On the other hand, these two types of organizations have contradictory atmospheres (that is, bureaucracies stress, for example, contractual, impersonal, instrumental relations while the family stresses the opposite), so moving them too close together would also make the job more difficult. Given these polar forces, the balance theory would suggest that the best way of handling most problems is to produce a relationship between the bureaucratic organization and the community primary groups that is balanced at some midpoint.

Policy Implications

To clarify this formulation, the three theories will be reviewed with regard to their policy implications. The separatist would, perhaps, keep the social worker and the client in the professional's office, isolated as much as possible from the community. The integrationist would argue that the community and the professional should be moved as close together as possible. The balance theory would suggest that the policy-maker assess the situation to determine whether the two groups are too far apart, in which case they should be moved closer, or too close together, in which case they should be moved farther apart.

The first two positions have by far the lesser burden in making a community diagnosis, for regardless of the diagnosis their policy is clear. In contrast, the policy-maker utilizing the balance theory could come to diametrically opposed conclusions depending on his diagnosis. Since situations change radically, it is quite possible that at one point in time the balance theorist would be advocating an integrationist program, while at another time he would be advocating one that is like the separatist. Thus, historically social workers dealt with social problems and worked in the community. At that point the balance theory would have sensitized the practitioner to the dangers of becoming too involved in the community. The turn to psychoanalysis led to a separatist point of view and the balance theory would suggest sensitivity to the problem of being too isolated. With regard to the current integrationist push, the balance theory would again suggest a sensitivity to the problems of excessive closeness. As will be shown, the theory does more than just suggest: it indicates in great detail the types of linkages that can be used to implement each formulation.

Optimal Functions of Organizations and Primary Groups

Before these linkage theories are explored, an attempt will be made to provide the theoretical underpinning for the balance theory—i.e., that formal organizations (professionals) and primary groups are both necessary for the achievement of most tasks even though they have contradictory atmospheres. A full understanding of this theory provides general guidelines for determining what tasks can best be handled by professionals, what can best be handled by nonprofessionals, and what fall in between.

To start the analysis extreme instances will be dealt with, and once the point has been made it will be shown how it can be generalized to intermediary situations. Discussion will begin with the polar forms of the bureaucratic organization and the family as a primary group, even though many people have pointed out that such organizations are not necessarily the best for contemporary industrial society. The reader need only keep in mind that they are useful because they are at opposite ends of the organizational continuum and the theory, once developed for the extremes, can quickly be generalized to intermediate cases.

Characteristics of Monocratic Bureaucracies

If one examines monocratic bureaucracies as defined by Weber, one can see why he made the claim that these are the most effective form of organization in an industrial society, for they clearly provide an organizational base for the maximization of knowledge.[9] First, they select and promote people on the basis of ability and knowledge, thereby ensuring that the most knowledgeable people are available. Second, they emphasize specialization, which ensures that the most knowledgeable people have an opportunity to develop and practice their knowledge. Third, they insist that relations within the organization be impersonal to prevent the introduction of personal likes and dislikes into the decision-making process and thereby ensure that knowledge and organizational tasks will be the pre-eminent bases for decision-making. Fourth, they insist on a priori definition of duties and privileges to ensure that people do not use their power within the organization to further personal goals. Finally, they provide two co-ordinating procedures to ensure that in this large organization the right person is performing the right task at the right time: (1) The use of general rules, which ensures that the entire organization will utilize common decision-making policies that neatly dovetail with each other, even when they are not in direct face-to-face contact. Written rules are a quick and efficient way of co-ordination when decisions can be anticipated ahead of time. (2) A hierarchical ladder of authority, which, when the situation is idiosyncratic, ensures that once a decision is made on an ad hoc basis all parts of the organization will be governed by a common decision.

Primary Group Characteristics

It is thus clear why this specific type of organization was thought to be so powerful, especially when compared to a primary group. The primary group is characterized by a stress on positive affect

---

[9] Gerth and Mills, eds., *op. cit.*

rather than impersonal relations: One is supposed to do things for people because one loves them, regardless of their abilities. Thus a father who leaves his business to his son frequently does so not because the son is the most able person to run it but because he loves his child and wants to do something for him. The primary group stresses noninstrumental relations. Even if one does not love a primary group member, one must preserve family ties as an end in itself. A father who does not especially love his son might still leave his business to him because he values family continuity. A parent will not disown or disassociate himself from a child who does not do well occupationally, because preserving the relationship is important in its own right.

Furthermore, the primary group does not stress specialization, but rather the opposite—diffused relations. In the family almost any area is a legitimate topic for discussion: religion, politics, education, leisure activities, and so on. Nor is there any a priori way (comparatively speaking) to delimit duties and obligations. Thus one family member may call on others for help in almost any circumstance.

The primary group also stresses the permanence of the relationship. It is true that there are instances of divorce, but these only partially remove the person from the family (especially if young children are involved) and it must be remembered that there are more institutional blocks to divorce than to the breaking of most other types of relations. Finally, primary groups stress face-to-face contact. This means that they must be small and therefore do not have a large enough population base for developing specialists or utilizing large-scale capital goods. It is now clear in what sense the bureaucratic organization seems a superior base for utilizing trained, knowledgeable persons.

When Is Expertise Not Necessary?

Given the fact that one of the chief advantages of the bureaucracy is its ability to produce trained experts, the question must be asked: When are trained experts not necessary for accomplishing tasks? It will be under such circumstances that the primary group is likely to play a role. The answer to this question is in part obvious. Expertise is of little use in at least three situations: (1) when the task is simple enough for the ordinary individual to do it as well as the expert, (2) when there is no knowledge base in which to train experts, and (3) when the situation is so complex or unexpected that a professional's knowledge cannot be brought to bear in time. These three instances will be referred to here as nonuniform events. If this point can be elaborated to show that such tasks constitute important areas of life and if in addition it can be shown that primary groups are more effective types of organizations when expertise is not necessary, then one component of the theoretical base for the balance theory will have been stated.

1. *When the average individual can do as well as the expert—* for example, in dressing children, providing daily meals, driving a car, buying clothes—in short, the everyday activities that comprise a considerable part of one's life. Experts may intervene in the family when for some reason the primary group has broken down. However, their intervention should involve an attempt to rebuild the primary group or to replace it with another primary group, for example, to help a mother become a better one or to find a foster home for her child rather than utilize a bureaucratic institution like an orphanage.

2. *When knowledge is so sparse that experts cannot be trained.* For example, in discussing everyday child-rearing practices that lead to the development of moral autonomy, a prominent researcher pointed out that there are so many gaps in our knowledge that it is difficult, if not impossible, to provide expert advice in this area.[10] Similarly, it can be pointed out that volunteers frequently do almost as well as professionals in such areas as treatment of alcoholism, overweight, narcotic addiction, and so on.

3. *Situations that are so unexpected or so complex that the expert's knowledge cannot be brought to bear quickly enough to make a difference.* Thus a mother might have to make a decision as to whether her 12-year-old daughter can sleep at a friend's house. This decision has a host of contingencies—it is a school

---

[10] Lawrence Kohlberg, "Development of Moral Character and Moral Ideology," in Martin L. Hoffman and Lois W. Hoffman, eds., *Review of Child Development Research* (New York: Russell Sage Foundation, 1964), esp. pp. 423 ff.

night and the daughter might not get enough sleep, the daughter
has been feeling left out and needs to develop closer relationships
with friends, the mother does not know the parents of the friend
and does not know if the children will be properly chaperoned, and
so on. In short, this simple decision has a host of contingencies
and must be made immediately. The day is continually filled with
such decisions and delay would slow down interaction far too
much. If the mother were to consult a professional about each such
decision, he would have to devote full time to this family alone,
which would result in a scarcity of professionals. Alternatively, if
the professional cannot be given all the pertinent information, his
decision will be no better than the mother's; that is, his greater
knowledge of psychodynamics is canceled by his lack of knowledge
of the facts in the specific case.

It is the author's contention that when the primary group and the
bureaucratic organization have equal knowledge, the former is
structurally a more efficient form of organization because it permits faster and more flexible decision-making as well as being less
expensive. The very aspects of its structure that make the primary
group defective in the production of trained experts make it efficient when trained experts are not needed. In contrast, the very
aspects of bureaucratic structure that enable it to produce trained
experts make it inflexible and slow when these are not needed.

To make this point clear, let us assume that we are dealing
with problems that do not require trained experts. The first advantage of the primary group is obvious. Special time and effort
are required to train experts and as a consequence specially trained
persons are in limited supply. In comparison, all people are members of a primary group. If a primary group can handle the problem almost as well as the expert, then just in terms of coverage and
cost it pays to have the primary group do it.

In addition, primary groups provide speedier and more flexible
decisions when nonuniform events are involved. Why is this so?
The primary group is a small organization with continuous face-
to-face contact among all members. Granted it has the same
knowledge as the bureaucratic organization, its face-to-face continuous contact permits more rapid feedback. This is especially
true when nonuniform events are involved in which there is a

lack of knowledge or that deal with complex or unanticipated problems. In such instances the bureaucracy must channel information through several levels of authority. Furthermore, the stress of primary groups on diffused relations is one of the factors that permit the face-to-face contact to be continuous. The stress on permanent relations means that people can learn the group's communication quirks and thereby utilize subtle cues to transmit information quickly; positive affect means that people are quite likely to trust each other and have a positive set toward messages, avoiding problems of selective listening and selective interpretation.

For many of the same reasons, the primary group is more flexible than the bureaucratic organization. This is especially apparent when dealing with areas in which there is no knowledge base. In such situations it is necessary to have an organization that permits a wide search operation. The primary group's legitimation of diffused relations, as compared to the bureaucratic organization's, provides for a wide intake policy. Finally, insofar as lack of knowledge leads to feelings of uncertainty, there is good reason to believe that positive states of affect are more functional for communication and work motivation than impersonal relations.

To sum up, the very structure of the primary group makes it more effective than bureaucratic organizations for dealing with nonuniform events. If this principle is followed and detailed, it can provide the social worker with a general policy for saying what tasks should be assigned to the professional and what should be assigned to the community. However, before beginning this most significant task, it is necessary to move from the use of these extreme cases to the intermediary situations, for much of what social workers deal with has to do with tasks that are mixed.

Degrees of Nonuniformity and Varieties of Organization

Any given task might be located on a continuum of uniformity to nonuniformity. The situation is a little like differentiating night from day at dusk and dawn: it is difficult to say at exactly what point one begins and the other ends, but nevertheless one would not argue that there is no difference between the two. The reader should keep this analogy in mind when dealing with the problems of classifying events as uniform or nonuniform. On the one extreme, it can be argued that some tasks are predominantly uniform, for example, licensing of automobile drivers. For the most part this can be routinized, various machinery can be used to expedite matters, and the small amount of nonuniformity can be handled via ladders of authority. One could similarly classify the billing activities of most utility companies, which can be standardized and handled through the expert as embodied physically in computers. Social security and many public welfare programs fit this model. Thus many public welfare programs for which social workers are hired in fact turn out to involve routine tasks. In all such cases it could be suggested that the most effective type of organization is the Weberian bureaucracy or a rules-oriented organization.

Tasks that are a greater mixture of nonuniform and uniform are those involved in activities such as psychotherapy or research. In each case a great amount of training is necessary. However, there is also a considerable amount of idiosyncratic behavior. Thus a research physicist may need a tremendous amount of training to know what it is that is unknown. Yet dealing with the unknown is a crucial aspect of his work. Similarly, a social worker needs a tremendous amount of training to do therapy, but the complexity of each case is so great that for all practical purposes substantial parts of the job have to be treated as unique events. If the balance theory is correct, this would mean there are pressures to have some combination of bureaucratic and primary group organizations. Such organizations do in fact exist and have been referred to in social work as offering a therapeutic milieu, in industry as goal-oriented or human relations organizations, and in other contexts as democratic or collegial organizations. As one moves to increasingly nonuniform tasks, it would be the writer's hypothesis that the organization that is most ideally suited to achieving these tasks approaches the true primary group. Thus we would posit an organizational continuum moving from the bureaucracy that Weber talks about through the collegial bureaucracy to forms of voluntary-professional organizations to voluntary organizations to informal clubs to primary groups.

The problem of classification is further complicated by the fact that the organization may wittingly or unwittingly have multiple tasks or tasks with clearly identifiable and separable components. For instance, a school has to provide motivation for the children— an area in which knowledge is minimal—and at the same time must maintain records of the child's attendance, how well he is doing, what subjects he has passed, and so on. Maintenance of such records requires large-scale facilities and the trained expertise that goes into their construction and use. Here are two clearly separable aspects. The situation is similar for hospitals: The doctor's analysis and treatment may be highly idiosyncratic while the maintenance of hospital records and the preparation of food for staff and patients are uniform events. If such organizations (when they have both uniform and nonuniform components that are clearly separable) are examined, they may be seen actually to have a dual system of adminstration (i.e., one part that deals with the uniform matters and is run like a Weberian bureaucracy and the other aimed at nonuniform matters and being run as a collegial bureaucracy).[11]

Perhaps this point might be made more dramatically in closed institutions. These may be institutions whose major goal is uniform, but which in order to be achieved demands full-time staff commitment. As a consequence the organization finds itself in the position of meeting all the nonuniform demands as well. Thus members of a submarine crew may have a highly programmed and technical mission that by all measures would be considered predominantly uniform. Yet by virtue of the fact that the men live on the submarine twenty-four hours a day for several months at a time, they must in turn deal with the nonuniform tasks as well. A similar situation exists in mental hospitals and prisons. Thus if the balance theory is correct, closed institutions must program for primary groups whether they want to or not.

A clear case in point of an attempt systematically to program and utilize the primary group as part of the treatment process is the

---

[11] Eugene Litwak, "Models of Bureaucracy Which Permit Conflict," *American Journal of Sociology*, Vol. 67, No. 2 (September 1961), pp. 177–184.

work done at Highfields.[12] This was a form of guided group interaction in which the inmates of Highfields, a training school for
delinquent boys, formed a continuing group. The norms of the
group encouraged antidelinquent behavior and complete honesty in
all statements about current and past behavior, there was no punish-
ment by formal authorities for things revealed in the group, and
the peer group decided whether a trainee was really ready to be
released. To the greatest extent possible the peer group was to do
the work of changing the delinquent behavior of inmates.

This must be contrasted with the ordinary prison process in
which a relatively innocent prisoner is left to the spontaneous primary group with its delinquent norms and will often emerge as a
hardened criminal—testimony to the effectiveness of the primary
group and to the fact that the prison organization does not fully
understand why such groups are more efficient than the bureaucracy in handling many problems. If authorities understood this
point in principle, they would move to a more explicit way of dealing with problems, as was done at Highfields.

There is yet another important instance when an organization's
multiple goals force it to deal with problems that it may not be
designed to handle. For instance, there may be a difference between long- and short-term prognosis. Thus psychiatrists may not
be able to deal effectively with the general problems of mental
health. Their procedures are frequently long and costly and the
probability of cure is low—consulting a psychiatrist may in many
areas be little better than going to a nonprofessional. Yet society
may still encourage psychiatry because it might feel that in the
long run that profession is likely to produce some meaningful in-
novation that will lead to a better cure. This is surely the kind of
bet society has made with all of science. In effect, society has said
a long-term goal should have precedence over a short-term one
and as a consequence the organization must deal with nonuniform
problems. If the balance theory is correct, in such cases the best
organization would be one that approaches the therapeutic or
collegial model. More generally, it should be pointed out that
costs are based on the probability of an organization's accomplish-

---

[12] H. Ashley Weeks, *Youthful Offenders at Highfields* (Ann Arbor: University of Michigan Press, 1958).

ing a task and how much it values this task. Thus it might be argued that even if use of psychoanalysis is costly it is still worthwhile, because our values suggest that anything that reduces the incidence of mental illness is important, no matter what the cost.

Without trying to exhaust the problem of classification, the general point being made should be clear. Primary group structures are ideal for handling nonuniform tasks. If the task has two separable components (one uniform and one nonuniform), then two types of organization are ideal—bureaucratic and primary group. If the task has two components that cannot be separated, then a mixed type of structure (e.g., collegial bureaucracy) is hypothesized to be ideal.

Technology and Classification of Events

The problem of classification is further complicated by the fact that technology might change certain tasks from nonuniform to uniform and vice versa. In fact, some would argue that technology will reduce all nonuniform events and that is why we must inevitably move toward a policy of bureaucratic organizations and lack of community interaction. If this is true, the separatist philosophy would be justified in the long run.

A close look at technology indicates how it has taken family tasks and shown how they can be better handled by trained experts: the development of commercial laundries, medical centers, clothing manufacturers, and modern communications media, for example, is ample testimony. However, when one moves away from the initial stages of technology and looks at the more advanced states, a different picture emerges. Thus in principle there is no reason why technology cannot take complex tasks and simplify them so the ordinary citizen can handle them (an example is development of home appliances).

The same line of reasoning can be pointed out for the other two aspects of nonuniformity, i.e., lack of knowledge and complex or idiosyncratic events. Thus scientists have pointed out that they do not necessarily reduce the area of ignorance even when they advance knowledge. This seeming paradox is true because with each advance in knowledge new areas of ignorance are found of which there had been no previous awareness. Thus technology produced an atomic bomb, which had unpredicted consequences in the area of international relations; introduced the automobile and found itself confronted with problems of air pollution and traffic safety. The dimensions of these problems could not be predicted before these inventions were made. Scientific advances are as likely to show things are more complex than was originally thought as they are to reduce one type of complexity to a predictable event.

The reader might think that what is being said is a philosophical point without much substance. However, one economist has estimated that the American family controls over $70 billion in investments, while industry controls only $50 billion.[13] This is a good measure of how much has in fact been returned to the family by technology.

If technology takes things away from the family as well as puts them back, what is the point? The point is that in principle it can do either. There is nothing in the logic of technology that says a family will have no meaningful tasks. What is suggested is more of a partnership with bureaucratic organizations, with each continually changing its functions as a consequence of technology but without either necessarily gaining or losing—after the initial stage of imbalance has been corrected. This analysis therefore suggests that the balance theory might well be supported by technological developments, i.e., primary groups in any conceivable future will always be better suited to doing some kinds of jobs.

Linkage Theory

At this point, let us briefly review the logic of this presentation. The argument has been made that bureaucratic organizations (and the professional) are best able to handle uniform tasks—those in which expert knowledge is needed—and that the primary group can best handle nonuniform tasks. The argument has been further made that technology will not fundamentally alter this fact. However, the point has also been made that the atmospheres of the

---

[13] Personal communication to the author by Bertram Gross, January 1967.

formal organization and the primary group are antithetical, which is the reason they can handle different tasks so effectively. If they were not antithetical, the integrationist point of view would be acceptable. As things now stand, however, it is the balance theory that seems most reasonable. The only question that remains to be answered is how linkages between community and bureaucracy can be programmed so as to keep the two close enough to work together while still sufficiently far apart to avoid problems of nepotism and favoritism within the bureaucracy or excessive contractualism and expediency within the community primary groups. Therefore, attention will now be turned to a subsection of balance theory that will henceforth be referred to as linkage theory.

As a first effort in developing this linkage theory, some procedures by which organizations typically relate to the community will be specified. No claim is made that these specific linkage procedures cover all possibilities or that they are exclusive (they can be used in combination). Their only virtue is that they are frequently used and as such serve as common bases for communication. If their underlying bases can be examined, then it should be possible to indicate how the social worker can develop entirely new procedures or to show that procedures that are apparently different really have the same underlying characteristics. With this in mind, the following eight empirical procedures will be defined:

1. *Detached worker.* A professional worker is sent outside the organization to the locale of the group the agency seeks to reach, and through establishment of a close, friendly relationship produces change. In its extreme form this is manifested by the youth gang worker who works with a gang in its home environment. Aggressive casework might also use this approach; examples in other areas are religious missionaries and possibly farm extension workers.

2. *Decentralized services.* These exist when agencies move their physical facilities as close as possible to their clients. This procedure differs from use of the detached worker in that the agency's facilities are physically present in the neighborhood and the professional does not leave the technical boundaries of the organization. The client must still come to the professional, al-

though he does not have as far to go. A typical example is the settlement house. The more contemporary concept of storefront services indicates an even greater decentralization than was the case with the settlements. This approach has been utilized in areas other than social work, such as the use of schools for after-school community programs.

3. *Opinion leader.* When the professional works through local indigenous leaders, it is called the opinion leader approach. The heavy stress on indigenous leaders in current antipoverty programs reflects this trend. In the area of consumer behavior, it has been argued that opinion leaders play a crucial role in determining the consequences of mass media.[14] Shaw and McKay made similar suggestions with regard to the treatment of delinquency.[15] One of the more significant works pointing out the problems of utilizing indigenous or local leaders has been presented by Selznick in his analysis of the Tennessee Valley Authority.[16]

4. *Local voluntary association.* In order to communicate with their community, organizations frequently work closely with voluntary associations, which may have an official or semiofficial status in the organization. Thus community chest or health foundation fund-raising drives frequently work through an extensive network of voluntary associations. Classic in this regard are parent-teacher associations in schools, lay clubs for churches, veterans' organizations, and hospital Gray Ladies. The central idea is that the voluntary association acts as a communication channel between the professional and the community.

5. *Common messenger.* When a person is a member of both the community primary group and the bureaucratic organization, he is called a common messenger: He can pass messages by virtue of his common membership in both groups. In some sense all people who work and have families are common messengers.

---

14 Elihu Katz and Paul F. Lazarsfeld, *Personal Influence* (Glencoe, Ill.: Free Press, 1955), pp. 1–100.
15 Saul Kobrin, "The Chicago Area Project: A Twenty-Five Year Assessment," *Annals of the American Academy of Political and Social Sciences,* Vol. 322 (1959), pp. 19–37.
16 Philip Selznick, *TVA and the Grass Roots* (Berkeley and Los Angeles: University of California Press, 1949).

This linkage procedure is perhaps the most dangerous in that it can most easily lead to conflict between the bureaucracy and the community primary group. As a consequence it is generally severely hedged in by role definitions. This approach currently is best seen in the stress on employing indigenous persons in antipoverty programs. The public schools make heavy use of this approach insofar as they send messages home with the child.

6. *Mass media.* When individuals use mass media such as radio, television, newspapers, mass meetings, demonstrations, leaflets, mass mailings, and the like to carry a message, it will be called a mass media approach. Although these means vary somewhat from each other, they have much in common.

7. *Formal authority.* The use of legal force or the threat of sanctions of some kind when used in conjunction with any of the methods cited will be called formal authority. Thus welfare workers have used threats of withdrawing aid as a way of communicating to the client that he must comply with the agency's regulations and schools employ truant officers who can use threats of legal proceedings to assure school attendance of minor children.

8. *Delegated function.* Finally, an organization can seek to reach a population by going through another organization that may already have access to it. Delegated function must always be used with one of the other mechanisms cited—that is, the organization contacted must reach its clients through one of these mechanisms. The problem of interorganizational relations will not be dealt with in this paper, which is restricted to direct contact with people.

With these empirical types of links before us, let us now turn to the theoretical dimensions that underlie them. We are interested in theories that say something about the power of these mechanisms to close the distance between the organization and the community.

Selective Listening and Organizational Initiative

Those working in the field of mass media have done much empirical work on the problems of bureaucratic organizations and community distance. They have pointed out in a variety of areas (e.g., consumer research, voter research, psychological warfare) that the key problem facing a bureaucracy trying to close distance with the community is selective listening.[17] People are predisposed to listen only to those messages with which they agree. Thus Democrats generally listen to speeches by Democratic candidates, people disposed to education are most likely to listen to messages that seek to develop educational involvement, people most hostile to Communism are those most likely to listen to anti-Communist propaganda, and so on. Because these researchers concentrated on only the mass communications media they tended to think in terms of various manipulations of those media—message content, status of message-giver, and so on.

However, if the list of mechanisms is re-examined, it quickly becomes apparent that there is a major organizational component that these researchers overlooked. This dimension will be referred to as organizational initiative. What is meant is that some of these linkage procedures clearly give the initiative to organizations as far as making sure the message is heard, while others give the initiative to the community primary groups. This initiative, in turn, is a major factor in determining whether a message will be heard. For instance, it is clear that mechanisms such as the detached worker and formal authority give the initiative to the organization, while mass media and opinion leader give it to the client. In the case of the detached worker, the professional is told to go to the client and stay with him until he gets the message. In the use of formal authority, the organization forces the client to listen by virtue of its power. By contrast, a person watching television can easily change channels if he does not like a program.

It is clear that the less an organization wants to communicate with the client, the more it should stress linking mechanisms that put the responsibility for communication on the client. If this analysis can be accepted, then it would seem that one essential dimension underlying all linking mechanisms is the extent to which they give organizational initiative to the client or the organization. In Table 1 the eight mechanisms are evaluated by their underlying dimensions.

---

[17] Herbert H. Hyman and Paul Sheatsley, "Some Reasons Why Information Campaigns Fail," *Public Opinion Quarterly*, Vol. 11, No. 4 (Fall 1947), pp. 412–423.

Table 1. Linking Mechanisms and Basic Dimensions for Dealing with Social Distance

Type of Linking Mechanism	Organizational Initiative	Primary Group Intensity	Focused Expertise	Scope
Detached worker	Highest	High	Highest	Lowest
Decentralized service	Moderate-low	High	High	Moderate
Opinion leader	Low	High	Low	Moderate
Voluntary association	Low	Moderate-low	Moderate-low	Moderate-high
Common messenger	Moderate	Moderate	Low	Moderate
Mass media	Lowest	Lowest	Lowest	Highest
Formal authority	Highest	Low	Moderate	Moderate
Delegated authority [a]	Any	Any	Any	Any

[a] In this mechanism the ultimate impact depends on which mechanism is used by the organization to which the function is delegated.

Selective Interpretation and Primary Group Intensity

Investigators in communications research have pointed out that overcoming the problem of selective listening is not sufficient to change a person's point of view. Even with a captive audience there is the problem of selective interpretation. Thus it is pointed out that language is sufficiently ambiguous that it can generally be reinterpreted to fit prior points of view.[18] Frequently cited as an example is the question: "Why did you buy this book?" This seemingly straightforward question has several different interpretations: why you bought it rather than stealing or borrowing it, why you bought a book rather than a sweater, or why you bought it rather than someone else. When the message is more complex, the problems of selective interpretation increase enormously.

In this regard, students of mass media have suggested that to ensure proper interpretation of a message it is best to have face-to-face contact to permit immediate feedback if the respondent misinterprets, the relationship must be one of trust so the respondent will give credence to the message-giver, and the relationship should follow the respondent in all areas of life so he does not compartmentalize it (refuse to see its relevance to other areas). The writer has referred to this kind of relationship as having primary group intensity because it seems to stress the same dimensions as the primary group—face-to-face contact, positive affect, and diffused relations. The argument would presumably be that the more primary group intensity a linking mechanism permits, the closer the social distance, while the less it permits, the greater the social distance. If the eight mechanisms are re-examined with this dimension in mind, it can be seen that two that were classified alike under initiative are now quite different. Thus the detached worker approach by definition should permit high primary group intensity. In contrast, according to most theorists formal authority tends to work against the development of high primary group intensity. Yet both of these mechanisms were rated as having high initiative.

Mass media follows still a third pattern. As contrasted to formal authority and the detached worker, it is rated as having low in-

---

[18] *Ibid.*

tensity as well as low initiative. The mechanism that has the most intensive relationship with the client is the opinion leader, because this is based on a natural primary group. However, it should be noted that the opinion leader, although linked to the community by intensity, is not necessarily linked to the professional or the bureaucracy by high intensity. His relationship to them may be quite impersonal, as suggested by studies of mass media. It is hypothesized in these studies that there is a three-step flow of communication from professional to mass media to opinion leader to client. Recognition that the opinion leader has this highly intensive relationship with the client has always been one of the reasons the local indigenous leader was considered to be the person through whom social workers should work. Such an approach overlooks two things, however: First, the social worker does not necessarily have strong ties with the opinion leader, and when the group is strongly deviant the leader may be the hardest person in the group to change. Second, when the task requires on-the-spot professional expertise, the opinion leader does not have the knowledge base. For this reason many social workers object to the area approach to delinquency developed by Shaw and McKay.[19] The eight mechanisms have been evaluated in terms of their primary group intensity under the column so labeled in Table 1.

Complex Messages and Focused Expertise

Messages can vary in the degree of their complexity and the extent to which it is necessary to have experts to provide answers. Thus messages that attempt to convey the time, place, and name of a speaker are relatively simple and unambiguous. In contrast, messages that seek to explain general philosophies of child-rearing or how to deal with the problems of a person who has been hospitalized for mental illness and is now returning home are complex. There is no simple standardized way to lay out a program.

Given the ambiguity of the message, it is necessary to have someone around to explain those aspects of the message that are unique for the case in point. This dimension differs from primary group

---

[19] *See* Kobrin, *op. cit.*

intensity in that it concentrates on the need for professional experts, while primary group intensity says nothing about expertise—it only stresses face-to-face, affective, and diffused relationships. It is suggested here that when individuals have complex messages that require expertise, to close social distance they should bring their experts in greater face-to-face contact with the client, and when they want to increase it, they should use such techniques as the mass media. In Table 1 each linking procedure has been rated according to this dimension.

Scope of the Mechanisms

Another dimension of communication often stressed has been called scope—how many people a mechanism can reach. Thus if people were equally receptive, it could be argued that the mass media have the widest scope. In contrast, the detached worker has the least, since he reaches but one group. This highlights one of the serious limitations of the detached worker program: It is costly in terms of personnel and money. Therefore, even though this may be a good strategy to use for decreasing social distance, it frequently cannot be used because of shortage of manpower or finances. On the other hand, when the client is favorably disposed and the message is relatively simple or can be made to appear simple, this form of linkage is extremely powerful.

Although there are other dimensions of linkage that must be examined, these are the ones, based on our current knowledge, that seem most pertinent to the problem of increasing and decreasing social distance. Properly handled, they can provide the base for a systematic theory of linkages for social work professionals as well as others who are interested in grass-roots organization.

Implications for Theory and Practice

The linkage mechanisms traced do not represent an exhaustive list. Each in fact has many variations. What the writer has done is provide an initial framework to evaluate all these variations plus any others one may come across. No matter what they are called, four things can be asked of them: how much organizational initiative they provide, how much primary group intensity they permit, how much focused expertise they permit, and how broad their scope is. When these questions are answered, one can assess their impact on social distance—whether they will close or open the gap between agency and community. These four propositions of linkage theory not only suggest ways for evaluating new techniques, but also suggest the type of inventions needed. A social worker knowing which underlying dimensions are necessary might now become sensitive to tailoring something completely new to fit his needs.

This approach not only permits evaluation and encourages invention, but in addition begins to suggest some more dynamic theory of linkages. Thus the fact that an approach like use of the detached worker is high on initiative and intensity but low on scope while the localized services are low on initiative, high on intensity, and moderate on scope suggests that these two procedures might be used in sequence for maximum effect in lessening social distance. The detached worker approach should be followed by the settlement house approach as quickly as possible. This sequencing in turn suggests types of problems that will emerge, for example, how a client is moved away from his more personalized detached worker to the localized service approach. The problem of sequencing becomes especially complex and important when the balance theory of co-ordination is the guiding theory, for here the social worker faces the problem of moving clients through a sequence of mechanisms depending on how successful they are in treatment. Thus when the worker has a client who is too distant, he must use high-initiative and high-intensity mechanisms, but the more successful he becomes the more he must use approaches that have moderate initiative and intensity. For clients who are too close, he might have to engage in the reverse sequence of mechanisms.

What is essential in this formulation is that these four dimensions—initiative, intensity, focus, and scope—provide basic building blocks that permit classification of linking procedures as well as development of the dynamic relationships among them. It should be clear that linkage theory, even though it is a subpart of balance theory, is relevant to both the separatist and integrationist positions, for in each case it suggests which forms of linkage will maximize the respective point of view. The full scope of the linkage theory cannot be developed here, partly because of limited space and partly because necessary basic research has yet to be done.

Grass-Roots Linkages to the Agency

Rather than go into great detail on any one part of this theory, the writer would like to sketch at least two other areas of major import for grass-roots organization. These involve the problems that confront practitioners when the grass roots seek to influence the organization. Up to now the writer has been speaking of how the professional working out of an organization influences primary groups. The other area that will be developed is the optimal organizational milieu for any given mechanism.

Upward Sequencing of Linkages

The problem of communicating from the grass roots to the organization is not quite the same as that of communicating to the grass roots from the organization. It is therefore necessary to devote separate attention to the former, which will often confront the grass-roots community organization practitioner. He may be the target of such an effort and would do well to understand it. Or, as frequently happens, grass-roots community organizers might find themselves representing a local neighborhood community seeking to change the policy of some bureaucratic organization, in which case they might face some difficulties if they sought to apply the analysis of linking procedures thoughtlessly.

One of the dimensions of linking mechanisms that makes little sense when operating from a bureaucratic base becomes crucial when operating from a primary group base—the availability of expert resources. In our economy this is best indexed by money. Thus if one examines each of the eight linking mechanisms, one finds that they are differentially weighted by the amount of professional resources or money required. For example, a detached worker implies a full-time professional. Whereas it is considered feasible for most bureaucratic organizations to hire such people to communicate with the grass-roots community, it would be problematic for a family to hire such experts to work with bureaucratic organizations.

This is similar to the use of localized services and mass media. It has been pointed out that when the audience is favorably disposed, the mass media can reach the largest number with the smallest per capita cost. However, it is sometimes important to recognize that absolute rather than per capita costs are important as well. Thus it does no good to tell a family that for as little as one cent per person one can reach 10 million people using television. It would be the rare individual family that would be in a position to put up $100,000 to use the mass media. Similarly, it is the rare family that can afford to set up its own physical facilities near a bureaucracy and hire professionals to deal with members of that bureaucracy. Although formal authority in its legal aspects is presumably open to all, in fact the amount of one's resources makes a difference. Thus the courts and the police are presumably concerned with protecting the individual family as well as the large corporation. However, corporations can hire private police and in court cases can employ several lawyers on a full-time basis, so that in fact they generally have an advantage over all but a few families.

In contrast to these linking mechanisms, some involve lower immediate costs to the family—the opinion leader, common messenger, and voluntary association. The former two require little effort because they are generally part of an ongoing social relationship. However, as used by the family, they are limited in scope.

For these reasons it is thought that the key to the initiation of communication from the grass roots to the formal organization is the local voluntary association. This requires little in the way of expert resources to create or maintain. Thus local neighborhood groups, mothers protesting the poor condition of schools, welfare recipients protesting cuts in grants, and the like can be formed with little resources other than the time of the people involved. The voluntary association is so close in structure to the primary group that setting up such an association and getting it running does not require specialized knowledge but can frequently be learned by primary group members on the spot. What differentiates the voluntary association from the opinion leader and common messenger is that, once formed, it provides a sufficiently large base for the hiring of professionals or the creation of physical resources. Thus a voluntary association of two hundred people might pool enough funds to hire an expert or give individual members free time to devote to the group's business.

If this analysis is correct, it can be suggested that there might be great differences in the way linking mechanisms are sequenced when they start from formal organizations as compared with community primary groups. In the first instance the organization has an option to start with any linkage, while in the second instance they might have always to start with the voluntary association and build from there.

The problem of sequencing is seen most clearly when primary groups and formal organizations are compared. However, a more precise statement would be one saying that the more resources a group has, the more options it has for sequencing, while the less resources it has, the more likely it will have to start its sequencing operations with voluntary associations. Thus it is possible that a poorer bureaucracy might find itself in a position similar to the family, while it is easy enough to point out a few spectacular cases of extremely wealthy families that could operate in ways similar to bureaucracies.

Differential Access of Organizations

It should be clear that unless the organization takes special precautions, mechanisms such as the opinion leader and common messenger will inevitably operate in any situation. If it is also recognized that positions of power in an organization are related to social class and that in the United States neighborhoods are also associated with social class, one is confronted with an interesting point—different neighborhoods systematically communicate with different parts of an organization. Middle-class families and neighborhoods have as their links with an organization that organization's leadership, while the working class has as its link the low-echelon personnel. When organizational decisions are made at the top of the organization, the middle-class primary groups have a distinct advantage, while the opposite would be true in the case of the working-class groups. On the other hand, when organizational decisions require close co-operation between the low- and high-echelon groups within it (and the outer community has contradictory views), it will result in conflict within the organization as well. The important thing to remember about upward communication is that when the organization takes no special precautions to deal with the community, linking mechanisms like the opinion leader and common messenger will invariably lead to the highest levels of most organizations receiving messages from the middle- or upper-class primary groups.

Organizational Vulnerability

Thus far the writer has spoken about dimensions of linking mechanisms. However, to understand fully the differential use of linking mechanisms when utilized by primary groups to influence bureaucracies, it is necessary to understand that most bureaucratic organizations are publicly exposed because of their size and the number of people who must co-operate for their existence. Furthermore, because they depend on public co-operation, they tend to have norms that are close to those of the dominant social group. When the message deals with the dominant social norms they can therefore be reached by linking mechanisms that do not have much initiative or intensity. In such cases all the primary group has to do is get the item into the newspapers and the bureaucracy will react.

Having made this point generally, it is important to introduce a serious qualification. Bureaucratic organizations have different degrees of vulnerability. For example, the mayor's office is much more vulnerable to public pressure the month or so before an election than it is a month after. Or bureaucracies directly linked to the public might be much more vulnerable to pressure than those that are linked indirectly, for example, retailers as contrasted with wholesalers.

This analysis was based on the assumption of a democratic community with individuals having relatively homogeneous values. However, if the community has sharply polarized groups with asymmetrical distribution of power, all that has been said about the accessibility of bureaucracies would apply only to the norms of the dominant group. With this in mind, the general point is that relatively passive linking mechanisms such as the mass media may have substantial effects when used by the grass roots against the organization. This analysis suggests a more general issue as to the constraints on linkage mechanisms imposed by organizational structure.

A brief summary of the problems of grass-roots attempts to influence bureaucratic organizations is in order. The fact that some of the linking mechanisms require professional resources means that for many situations the primary group is forced into a fixed sequence in reaching a bureaucratic organization—that is, moving from mechanisms that require less resources to those requiring more. In contrast, bureaucratic organizations can utilize almost any sequencing. Second, some mechanism—for example, the common messenger and opinion leader—will operate in all circumstances unless organizations make special efforts to stop them. When organizational leadership makes no special effort, the consequences will be that the low-income group will meet only the lower echelon of the organization and the high-income groups will meet the leadership. Finally, the point was made that because the organization is so dependent on public co-operation, it can frequently be reached by relatively passive low-intensity mechanisms such as the mass media. This would be increasingly true the more democratic the community, the more symmetrically power was distributed, and/or the more the issue dealt with dominant social norms.

Limitations of Organizational Structures on Linkage Procedures

This analysis could be carried on to point out that those communicating from the grass roots to the organization are further faced with the problem of knowing where to intervene to get the best results. Although the same problem technically exists for the organization trying to reach the family, it is not as important because organizations are much larger and have a more detailed division of labor.

This problem of where to intervene in the organization can be put into a more general framework and from the point of view of the organization as well. Thus one can ask what limitations are put on the use of linking mechanisms by the structure of their host bureaucratic organizations. Placing the discussion within the latter framework has the added advantage of suggesting to the policy-maker where he must change his structure if he hopes to utilize a given linkage procedure for reaching the community.

To highlight this point, let us look at the administrative styles of two types of bureaucracies, the custodial institution and the therapeutic milieu. The former resembles the Weberian monocratic structure in that staff are selected on merit, specialization is stressed, obedience to written rules and hierarchical authority is emphasized, and a priori delimitation of duties and privileges as well as impersonal relations are encouraged. In extreme contrast, an organization characterized as having a therapeutic milieu stresses generalization rather than specialization, internalization of organizational policy rather than use of written rules, a stress on collegial rather than hierarchical relations, movement toward positive affect among people in the organization rather than impersonal relations. This therapeutic bureaucracy is similar to the Weberian rationalistic model only in its stress on merit.

Given these two extremes of organizational structure, one might well ask if they put any restraints on the types of linkage that can be used. To get some insight into this aspect of grass-roots theory, the writer would suggest that initially a principle of consistency be advanced. Those linking mechanisms that are inconsistent with the bureaucratic structure are least usable in that structure. This now suggests an examination of the linkage mechanisms in terms of the amount of centralized or decentralized authority they require, the amount of impersonal or affective relations they require, and so on.

For instance, let us consider the detached worker approach as concretely manifested in a youth gang worker. Several things about this approach seem clear: The youth worker has to make many decisions on the spot; he cannot go back to his superior every time a decision has to be made. It is difficult if not impossible to write any but the most general rules governing his behavior. Each gang has its own unique problems and the social worker has to play each decision by ear. It is difficult, as a consequence, to set down ahead of time the duties and privileges of this position. It is difficult, for instance, to specify something as standardized as hours of work. In short, the detached worker is a linking mechanism that is much more consistent with the structure of the collegial bureaucracy than the rationalistic one suggested by Weber. This inconsistency, if not taken into account, can completely negate the efforts at linkage.

For instance, in one case a school had hired a community agent to act as a detached worker in its neighborhood. The generalized directive was to get the neighborhood residents into the schools—to use the after-school facilities—and to develop a more positive backing of the school by the resident. However, this program could never be implemented, because the principal ran his school in a rationalistic way. He insisted that the community agent get permission every time he left the building and that he also indicate where he was going. In addition, the community agent could make no commitments on his own. This meant that not only did the principal have to be consulted, but permission had to be gotten through official channels from the superintendent's office. When the community agent wanted to schedule a dance at the school, it took several months for this process to operate. The principal was not required to take this position, since his school was part of a special program. Other schools that were part of the same program did not operate this way. The imperative for running the school in this manner was the principal's limited understanding of what ideal administrative styles were. He literally had no concept of an alternative to his style. Similar problems have arisen in probation departments in which the goals of therapy demand much discretion on the part of the professional, but when legal requirements insist that the job be treated in a uniform and rationalistic way.[20]

The implications should be clear. To utilize linking mechanisms that require decentralized decision-making and highly personal involvement, one must have a bureaucracy with a therapeutic milieu. If the linking mechanisms are inconsistent with the bureaucracy, one of three things can happen: (1) The linking mechanisms will not be implemented or may exist in name only. (2) Alternatively, the organizational structure will change. Thus one of the unanticipated consequences of the adoption of a specific community linking procedure has been change in the administrative styles of the bureaucracy. To some extent, such a shift has occurred in probation departments. (3) Continual interpersonal conflict may exist between those serving the bureaucracy and those serving the linking mechanisms. This may go along with the covert and illegal implementation of various linking mechanisms. Typical in this regard was the reaction of social workers handling probation or public welfare cases who ignored explicit rule violation of the client because in their professional judgment rule obedience was secondary to social work treatment goals. This condonation of illegal behavior was accompanied by running hostility, withholding of information, and the like among members of the bureaucracy.

In contrast to mechanisms like the detached worker approach, there are others such as formal authority and mass media that can be run much more effectively from a rationalistic milieu. Insofar as the mass media seek to reach a large and common audience, it makes sense to have one co-ordinated effort rather than many overlapping ones. Thus hierarchical authority, specialization, and rules orientation make sense here. Expertise and the economies of large scale can be maximized in such a situation.

Up until now the writer has spoken about the implication of such a program for the policy-maker or the professional in the bureaucracy; the implications would be equally great for those in

---

[20] Lloyd E. Ohlin, Herman Piven, and Donnell M. Pappenfort, "Major Dilemmas of the Social Worker in Probation and Parole," in Zald, ed., *op. cit.,* pp. 523–528.

the grass roots seeking to reach a given bureaucracy. If one is dealing with a bureaucracy that has decentralized decision-making, the directive is to move into the lower echelon positions where the decision has been decentralized. As far as the rationalistic bureaucracy is concerned, decisions of any ad hoc kind or exceptions to the decision have to be made at the top. If it is a question of implementation of given rules, it may be strategic to go to the lower echelons again, depending on the level at which the grass roots have defined their problem. Also, rationalistic bureaucracies may be best reached through formal linking mechanisms while therapeutic milieu bureaucracies might best be reached through mechanisms that permit primary group intensity. Perhaps more important, this formulation should indicate to both the community primary groups as well as the professional that changes in community programming frequently cannot take place without radical implications for administrative style. As a consequence, it forces both parties to consider systematically where their problem lies—for example, in the linkage procedures or in the administrative structure. Furthermore, it suggests a host of alternatives. In Table 2 is a suggested rating of the various linking mechanisms in terms of their consistency with types of bureaucratic groups.

In the discussion thus far stress has been placed on the notion of consistency between linkages and bureaucratic organizations. The discussion is limited by the fact that there are more styles of organization than the two extreme ones mentioned. Since this paper is overly long, other alternatives will not be covered; a start has been made on this elsewhere.[21]

However, there is one aspect of organizational structure that must be mentioned because it points out that "consistency" is not being used in a narrow sense. It has been pointed out elsewhere that an organization may in fact have two contradictory systems running simultaneously (e.g., the rationalistic and therapeutic administrative styles) within its boundaries as long as it has internal

---

[21] Eugene Litwak and Henry H. Meyer, "Administrative Styles and Community Linkages," *Schools in a Changing Society* (New York: Free Press, 1965), pp. 53–73.

Table 2. Consistency of Linking Mechanisms with Dimensions of Organizational Structure

Linking Mechanisms	Authority Structure	A Priori Rules	Interpersonal Stress	Need for Professional Training
Detached worker	Decentralized	Internalized policy and minimal rules	Personal	Professional
Settlement house	Decentralized	Internalized policy and minimal rules	Personal	Professional
Opinion leader	Centralized when favorable and decentralized when not favorable	Rules when favorable and internalized policy when not	Impersonal when favorable and personal when not	Nonprofessional
Voluntary association	Moderately centralized	Moderate rules	Semipersonal	Semiprofessional
Common messenger [a]	Centralized	A priori rules	Impersonal	Moderate
Mass media	Centralized	A priori rules	Impersonal	Professional
Formal authority	Centralized	A priori rules	Impersonal	Professional
Delegated function [a]	Centralized	Rules	Impersonal	Professional

[a] In the case of the common messenger and the delegated authority, there can in fact be tremendous variations. These specific ones have only been suggested as the way in which these linking mechanisms are most often used.

mechanisms of isolation.[22] Thus earlier in this paper the writer suggested that schools, hospitals, and many closed institutions must deal with the problem of tasks that have different demands and cannot be separated from each other. The reason these contradictory demands do not lead to disruption is the existence of mechanisms by which they are kept separate. Without trying to detail these mechanisms here, let it suffice to say they are analogous to role separation that permits a man to act in a contractual manner in his business relations and in a positive affective manner in his family relations. Thus when an organization has internal mechanisms of isolation, it is possible for it to tolerate several types of linking mechanisms simultaneously.

Summary and Conclusion

This now concludes the overall framework for the grass-roots balance theory of community organization. It should again be noted that such a theory provides only a partial answer to the problems of practitioners. It does not, for instance, say anything about some of the larger problems of community organization, for example, the relationship of organizations to each other. Its virtue is that it does deal with a clearly definable area of social work practice for which there has been little in the way of systematic theoretical guidelines. To make this point clear, a brief recapitulation of the major points of the theory has been presented in Table 3.

There are three major orientations toward grass-roots community organization. One, which has been labeled the separatist, states that the professional should not attempt any contact at all. Another, which has been called the integrationist, suggests just the opposite—the professional should merge with the local community. A third, which has been called a balance theory, suggests the professional should be at some midpoint of social distance from the community.

---

[22] Litwak, *op. cit.*

Table 3. Policy Implications of Three Theories of Grass-Roots Community Organization

Administrative Style	Linking Mechanisms	Separatist		Integrationist		Balance Theory	
		Deviant Families	Friendly Families	Deviant Families	Friendly Families	Deviant Families	Friendly Families
Therapeutic	High initiative and intensity	Lowest [a]	Lowest	Highest	Highest	Highest	Lowest
Rationalistic	Passive, low intensity	Highest	Highest	Lowest	Lowest	Lowest	Highest
Rationalistic	High initiative and intensity	Internal conflict	Internal conflict	Internal conflict	Internal conflict	Internal conflict	Internal conflict
Therapeutic	Passive, low intensity	Moderate	Moderate	Low	Low	Low	Moderate

[a] The rankings in this table refer to the columns. Thus in the first column for the separatist theory the highest ranked situation for handling deviant families is the rationalistic administrative style and the passive, low-intensity mechanisms. This would be the ideal that many administrators of income maintenance programs would hold.

The separatist point of view would in turn imply for all types of families—deviant or friendly—a rationalistic bureaucracy with formalistic linking mechanisms or a therapeutic bureaucracy with no community linking mechanisms. This is indicated in the left-hand column of Table 3, in which the "highest" designation is given to rationalistic organizations with passive low-intensity linking mechanisms. In contrast, the integrationist point of view suggests that the best solution for all types of families (both deviant and friendly) would be a therapeutic milieu with high-initiative and high-intensity mechanisms. Thus it can be seen from the middle column of Table 3 that this is the solution with the highest rating. Finally, if the column on the extreme right is examined—that designated the balance theory—it can be seen that the solution depends on the type of family. Thus, when the family is designated as deviant, the therapeutic milieu with high-initiative and high-intensity mechanisms is ranked highest; when the family is friendly, the rationalistic structure with the passive low-intensity mechanisms is ranked highest. This is, of course, a much simplified presentation of what has been said here. It must again be noted that limits of space prevented an even more detailed statement of the theory. Such a development is necessary to turn this analysis from a general orientation to a practice theory. However, even in this brief presentation it should be clear that this orientation lends itself to a more detailed specification. Whether or not the reader agrees with all of the specifics of even this abbreviated presentation, it is hoped that it is sufficiently suggestive to encourage future developments.

A social work approach to a mental health objective

Bertram M. Beck

Down through the years the social work approach to mental health objectives has been characterized by three basic tenets: (1) a theoretical construct or formulation about the problem under concern, (2) flexibility in the approach to problems, and (3) a concern with specific problems as opposed to general states or conditions. This paper will trace the development of these tenets from the profession's early concern with mental health to its present involvement in the War on Poverty.

History of the Social Work Approach

While social work at the turn of the century was responsive to the social conditions under which men lived and was rightfully concerned about the effect of these conditions on individuals, the

advent and popularization of Freudian psychoanalytic theory had
a great effect on the social work perspective on mental health problems. The tendency became to define these problems as intrapsychic.
Nevertheless, it was still recognized that the individual's environment has an effect on him and that a worker might as part of the
treatment process attempt to change his client's environment. In
actuality, however, since it was easier to work with a client's problems in adjusting to his environment than with changing the environment that caused these problems, the field's response to
problem-solving was essentially an individual psychological approach. The result was that workers ultimately were not dealing
with specific problems clients presented, but with individuals who
had problems. They were promoting an individual's adjustment
or mental health rather than specifically dealing with marital discord or delinquency. A subtle constraint to do this existed since
such problems as delinquency and marital discord are connected
with many other problems, both psychological and social. One
cannot simply cure a client's delinquency without dealing with
many other aspects of his life. Thus, while the social work profession always claimed—and with some justification—that it was
problem oriented, in reality its orientation was to the individual
client's adjustment on a broad level.

The social work profession has always accented the idea that in
grappling with a problem one must have some conceptual means
of understanding it. The difficulty social work has had in dealing
with problems of mental health is that while the need for theory
has long been known, an actual comprehensive social and psychological theory has not been developed. The number of articles
that end with the plea for more theoretical constructs is legion.
Yet it is difficult to fault the field for this lack of theory, since
perhaps more than any other of the helping professions it has at
least recognized the need.

This is apparent in the second tenet—flexibility. The social
work profession has always emphasized that the social worker
brings to bear on his client—whether an individual or a group—
economic theory, psychological theory, social theory, and the like.
The social worker draws on many different areas of knowledge to
deal with the problems with which he is concerned. The worker

has also been advised to be flexible in his use of techniques and methods, since ultimately what he does or fails to do is dependent on the needs of his clients. His specific treatment techniques are to be varied flexibly according to differential diagnosis.

In actuality the worker's flexibility has been severely circumscribed: (1) By theory or the lack of it—if caseworkers used psychoanalytic theory, then their flexibility was limited to the range permitted by that theory. (2) By the worship of professional training—if more personnel are needed to solve a problem, then the answer is to get more professional personnel rather than to inquire into the possibility of using other personnel with different kinds of training. (3) By agency structure—if agency procedures and policies called for a specific kind of service, only the rare social worker could alter these procedures.

An Expanded Approach

An intriguing factor about the three tenets cited is that their generality enables some practitioners to claim there is actually nothing really new about approaches to mental health problems that have been developed in the War on Poverty and the agencies connected with it. While it is true that the field has always had a flexible, theoretical, and problem-oriented approach, the boundaries of this approach have been significantly altered to the point at which the 1960s will most certainly be seen as a watershed in the development of social welfare in this country. For example, experience at Mobilization For Youth, a demonstration-research project on New York City's Lower East Side established for the control of juvenile delinquency, has led the agency's staff to certain conclusions concerning a social work approach to mental health.

First, a social work approach to mental health is best ordered when it is characterized by a definition of the kind of problem behavior a specific program aims to reduce or alter. One advantage of such an orientation is that it is easier to define a target population if one is addressing oneself to a specific kind of behavior manifested by a specific group of people. One is pushed to state the group to whom the services are being addressed, whereas to take the alternative, if one is addressing oneself simply to promotion of the good life it is easy to slip into the position of serving only those people who happen to come into the program, because there is no clearly defined target population: everybody is a candidate for the good life. Another advantage is that results are made somewhat more measurable. To an extent the increase or decrease of delinquency can be measured, but it is much more difficult to rate family stability or child development.

An added advantage of relation to a specific target population is that the agency's efforts and accomplishments can be scrutinized more easily and it can be held accountable in a more realistic sense by the community it serves. After all, one of the prime reasons agencies in the main—at least in the 1950s—withdrew from giving service to the poor was that it was possible under the guise of promoting the good life or good mental adjustment to deal only with those clients who were interested in the kind of treatment available. Thus the poor were not served.

Last and most important, a problem orientation forces programs to be specifically related to problem areas. Take for example an adult employment program. The target group is clearly the unemployed or those who wish to seek employment. The results will be measurable: How many unemployed people were helped to obtain employment? Casework services may be offered to mobilize clients' ego strength to seek employment; however, no attempt should be made to deal with general adjustment, family discord, or child neglect except to the extent that they impinge on a client's ability to seek and hold employment. This approach does not deny that clients may have much broader adjustment problems, but it does in a sense represent a form of accountability. It acknowledges both that a range of problems exists and that priorities must be set on the basis of what the community feels is important.

This conviction about the necessity of a problem orientation is related directly to MFY's second conclusion, that it is vital to have some theoretical construct about the nature of the problem that is being dealt with. Theory and practice must interact with one another; each grows from this interaction. While social work has in recent years borrowed heavily from the social sciences, the development of practice theory has not grown apace. There are a number of reasons for this. One surely is the fact that social work has not been as accountable as it might have been, that it has not defined its problems so that its solutions can be tested and measured to the greatest degree possible. Another and perhaps more important reason—one that is shared with all other professions—is that if one's major skill in working with clients is casework, one will tend to define problems in terms that allow one to use casework; if the law, then through legal techniques; and so on. Solutions tend to be defined by known techniques; the professional way becomes the right and only way and acts as a rationale for one's actions.

Opportunity Theory

MFY was fortunate in beginning its program with theoretical formulations supplied by Richard A. Cloward and Lloyd E. Ohlin.[1] Their concept of opportunity theory held essentially that delinquency in a ghetto is produced because neighborhood youngsters do not have the same access to legitimate means of gaining society's rewards as do youths in more favored neighborhoods. They contended that social institutions—school systems, welfare agencies, the police department, housing authorities, and the like—do not provide means for people in a ghetto to climb the social ladder and so become part of the larger society. Therefore in the ghettos there is a preponderance of delinquent behavior characterized by youths with thwarted legitimate aspirations who turned to illegitimate means of gaining status or material goods. Cloward and Ohlin suggested that if a program is to reduce delinquency, it must address itself to the malfunctioning of institutions and produce institutional change.

While this theory unfortunately was not completely operationalized by MFY, it did offer program directions. It suggested imparting skills—work, educational, and social—to the ghetto population so that they can gain organizational power, economic power, and individual security. The program focused essentially on the rela-

---

[1] *Delinquency and Opportunity: A Theory of Delinquent Gangs* (New York· Free Press of Glencoe, 1960).

tionship of individuals and the society of which they are a part. It was not the techniques that the workers possessed, it was not a general orientation toward promoting social integration, but it was a specific theory related to a specific social problem that guided MFY's programs.

Opportunity theory left many questions unanswered and did not completely lead MFY to the kinds of programs that would solve the problem of delinquency. Staff quickly found that it was necessary to be flexible in its use, as well as in the application of that part of it that seemed and proved to be useful. With regard to the problems of families in the area and their difficulties with welfare, housing, and the schools, opportunity theory suggested only in the most general way what should be done—make these institutions more responsive. In tackling the problem of making institutions more responsive MFY was aided by the fact that it had clearly defined a target group—the lower economic 10 percent of the population. In the absence of specific problem-related theory, focusing on a target group was a great help, since it confronted staff with the need for constant redefinition of method.

Evolution of an Approach

The first approach was to open neighborhood service centers, easily accessible storefronts where clients with welfare, housing, health, or legal problems could come for referral. The service centers were manned by trained workers who saw themselves as brokers who would direct people who lacked skills in manipulating bureaucratic structures to existing services. These centers were informal—with clients on a first-name basis with workers—and attempted to meet clients' needs through such means as providing a drop-in care center where mothers could leave their children while they kept clinic or other appointments.

The informality of the centers was well received and the agency was soon overwhelmed with clients. But workers found that their brokerage function was really not adequate. Despite their closeness to the neighborhood, MFY workers were no more successful when making referrals to the traditional agencies or public structures than others were. The problems of waiting lists, bureaucratic structure, and lack of sensitivity to the needs of the ghetto resident were just as great. It was clear that some new role for the worker would have to be developed—in truth it was developing all the time as workers increasingly advocated the needs of their clients before the various bureaucracies. (Advocacy is, of course, not necessarily a new role or one foreign to social work. Social workers have long seen themselves as partisans of their clients to some extent, even though this partisanship has been tempered by allegiance to the agency and the agency's allegiance to other social establishments.)

Advocacy produced many positive results for clients, yet focusing once again on the actual effect on the client group it was clear that this role itself created new problems. Staff were constantly dealing with problems such as welfare checks not arriving, emergency relief needed and not given, eviction notices, the arbitrary or discriminatory judgment of welfare investigators, and so on. These problems and the people who had them kept recurring. It was clear that staff were to an extent walking on a treadmill: institutional change was not being produced; the bureaucracy was merely being bent a bit. A redefinition of the problem was called for.

At this juncture the decision was to move from solely giving individual service to neighborhood organization. Staff began organizing groups of welfare clients with the idea that this might produce greater pressure on the welfare system than telephone calls by workers. This change proved to be in many ways quite successful; literally tens of thousands of dollars were recovered for members of these groups. Hundreds of people joined the welfare organizations, people who prior to this had never joined or participated in any organization. The groups also resulted in considerable growth of some individual members. Many leaders of these groups went on to enter work training programs and have left welfare assistance behind.

MFY has been led back, however, to its original problem of institutional change. Even under top leadership the welfare department cannot change quickly enough to respond to the realistic and reasonable demands of the organized clients—and not all the demands made are realistic and reasonable. The frustration of

the organized groups grows and it cannot be channeled or controlled by MFY staff or moderate leadership. Thus MFY, the
welfare department, and the clients are confronted by one facet
of the problem that currently besets America, namely, awakened
aspirations of exiled people without the social means for adequate
response.

Development of Practice Knowledge

This experience with the neighborhood service center illustrates
clearly that once a problem is confronted it constantly redefines
itself. Everything the agency did merely served to redefine the
problem and bring about further problems—which is the only way
progress is made. The organization of welfare clients together with
advocacy introduced certain dilemmas, the first, of course, being
whether a social worker can really maintain a stance of opposition
to the Establishment while being paid by it.

Today the climate is more permissive of this than ever before;
there is greater sanction for the idea that it is helpful for people to
speak up. The social worker has always had a kind of dual loyalty.
What MFY has done is point up this dilemma more sharply and
push the agency toward a greater allegiance to those without
power to advance social work or social workers but with the need
for social power themselves. It seems clear that the ultimate elim-
ination of poverty and the achievement of power for the target group
cannot be brought about through protest actions, even on a nationwide basis. Nevertheless MFY, by co-operating with the larger
social movement and abetting it, did so with the knowledge that
it presents an opportunity for the agency to learn and further redefine the problem in terms of its experience.

Another example of MFY's flexible, problem-oriented, and theoretical approach is in the field of community development. Here
the approach has been quite different from that characterized by
antipoverty programs that have placed great emphasis on board
membership for neighborhood residents. The latter approach is
characterized by a desire for the maximum feasible participation
of the poor. While there is nothing inherently wrong and obviously

much right with this orientation, it is not a problem orientation and has been fraught with problems. The MFY approach has been to bring people together around common specific problems as consumers, tenants, or members of minority groups. By organizing groups around specific issues or problems on an ad hoc basis, significant success has been achieved. In the neighborhood served by MFY at least thirty Puerto Rican, Negro, tenant, consumer, or welfare client organizations have developed, and these have grown to the point at which they often contend with MFY itself: that is, they have begun to seek—and get—money of their own from the antipoverty programs. MFY has also been flexible in its use of staff, hiring many local people as leaders. Staff have been permitted to take on a much more active role than is usually prescribed in traditional community organization work.

This flexibility has advanced the agency's thinking in terms of practice theory. It now seems that although development of mass organization around mass issues is a vital part of organizing a neighborhood, this must be followed by a second wave of organization—the organization of people having similar problems.

Whether or not this idea is correct, it illustrated the necessity of problem-solving within a theoretical formulation that is flexible in its search for new solutions. Without such an approach there will be no growth in practice. For example, advocacy must be defined just as other social work methods have needed definition. Lawyers take to advocacy in a way that social workers do not. Of course, this is their profession and their ethic. The rightness of seeking a change in law is clearly sanctioned by society even though change is painful.

MFY has learned a great deal about the value of advocacy for social workers. For example, the New York City Board of Education bars counsel in school suspension hearings. In other words if a child is to be suspended from school a hearing is held at which the child has no right to counsel. The reasons given for this are the right of confidentiality and protection of the child. The school authorities contend that suspension hearings are not punitive and are held to determine what action best serves the child's interests— the child needs no protection from the school system and therefore a lawyer is not needed for the hearing. Yet it is obvious that when a non-English-speaking mother attends such a hearing with her child she needs protection no matter what the school's intent is. MFY sought to obtain representation for children at suspension hearings by means of discussion and agitation, but without any success. It was then sought through the courts, but after success in the lower courts, the case was lost in the higher courts. Public attention, however, was focused on the issue and the MFY position gained many adherents. Ultimately a reconstituted Board of Education adopted the MFY position.

Few people will argue against taking a constitutional issue to the courts, but there will be much opposition when an attempt is made to raise a moral or procedural issue through discussion and consultation. Thus the advocacy method is quite important for social workers to master and the relationship of social work advocate to legal advocate must be furthered.

Summary

Out of the MFY experience a few specific conclusions were reached about a social work approach to mental health problems:

1. It is necessary to have some means of constantly monitoring the composition of the group being reached—that is, the income level, ethnicity, educational level, and the like—to provide for an immediate correction of program emphasis. There is a tendency in all programs, as problems are addressed and the attendant frustration met of failure to find adequate solutions, for the program to move toward the easiest target, toward people who can adapt themselves to the kinds of service or program being offered, thereby providing a spurious feeling of success.

2. There must also be some means of evaluating a program's success. While the potentiality of formal, rigorous research for evaluating programs must not be ignored, the difficulties of instituting such research should not lead the agency to overlook the value of simply finding out whether the clients like the program. The tendency in any profession is always to exercise its own judgment as to the merit of its activities. This is a crucial error.

3. In the use of personnel there must be flexibility but not romanticism. There can actually be no flexible approach to problems if there is no flexibility in the use of personnel. At MFY neighborhood residents without formal social work education have been used successfully in a variety of jobs—as vocational counselors, investigators in the legal program, social workers. Emphasis must be on what a person can do, not on what his educational credentials are. This will require specification of just what a job function is rather than definition of a job by the necessary educational qualifications. The agency must also provide means of on-the-job training for the development of all personnel.

4. One final trap must be cautioned against. Even with flexibility, problem orientation, and theoretical constructs, organizations may still develop rigidities that tend to impede their ends. Staff had to discover that MFY itself is a large bureaucracy that often does not serve its clients' needs. Commitments to specific programs grow, one part of the organization does not communicate with another, clients are confused by its size—as are the staff—and people have different ideas about how things should be done and different priorities about what should be done. MFY has thus been forced to redefine and reappraise its total service structure. The trap to be avoided is an overemphasis or focus on any one program. To the extent possible a social service organization should see itself as a total institution wherein all the programs and personnel are so structured that they sustain the agency's end.

Deviant roles and social reconnection

Elliot Studt

Out of ten years' exploration of problem areas in the correctional field have emerged some ideas about social work practice in that field that have possible relevance for social work practice in the field of mental health in general. Although the writer's work has been limited to public agencies dealing with offenders after they have been officially identified and committed, and so does not have immediate relevance for preventive treatment, it is clear that the principles of action developed in the prison experiment described in this paper are generally transferable to work in a field service. Important adaptations in service design will, however, be required by factors characteristic of work in the open community that are different from those operating in an institution.

The Client's Task

In analyzing a field of social work practice the question asked first determines the direction of the analysis and its outcome. The most fruitful opening approach when attempting to discover the potential role of social work in the correctional process is: What is the client's task?

Starting the analysis with questions about the client's task deliberately sets aside the medical analogue as a model for examining social work practice. The writer is not seeking to define a disorder to be treated by an expert in pathology. Rather, concern is with identifying the adaptive tasks created by the need for fit between the individual and his social environment that each person in a specific client population must resolve in some way, with or without help. "Adaptive task" is similar to what is meant when one says "the client's problem," but does not make the assumptions of primary personal inadequacy that are usually implied by that formulation.

The correctional client's task may be usefully conceptualized as an especially difficult form of a common human task generally known as a "status-passage." All of us live through a succession of status-passages as we grow and change in relation to our social environment. We move from "child-at-home" to "student-in-school," from hospitalized sick person to life in a normal setting, from married person to widowed, from beginning employee to supervisor. In every such process the individual is presented with a life task requiring some transformation in his personal and social identity, with all that such an adaptation can mean for the breakup of old patterns and the establishment of new.

Each convicted offender (except for those few who spend the rest of their lives in prison) must make the social and psychological transition from a publicly degraded status as a criminal deviant to the status of free person in the community if he is to be successful in either his or the community's terms. This task involves a double transformation of identity, first to that of convicted offender and then to a reconstitution of self as a normally functioning member of the community. A short way to describe the correctional client's life task is to say that he must achieve social reconnection from the position of an officially labeled deviant.

In most status-passages a transitional period between one status and the next is commonly recognized either formally or informally, providing for that period a supporting set of protections, opportunities for trial-and-error experimentation, and phased goals. Thus we generally accept *engagement* as a transitional step from the status of single person to that of married person, *bereavement* as a period between the married role and the reorganization of activities in the widowed role, *convalescence* as an important phase between a critical illness and the full assumption of normal role obligations, *probation* as a beginning period for the new supervisor, and some sort of *apprenticeship* as a planned transition leading to the exercise of professional responsibility. Such transitions permit both the individual and those around him to revise their expectations and customary behavior as needed to complete the psychological and social adaptations implicit in any transformation of identity. In the case of the correctional client, the entire correctional process can be usefully understood as one of these transitional periods, often involving distinct phases. During the correctional transition both the offender and his community can, under controlled conditions, test each other out, practice new relationships, and seek to establish the reciprocal interactional patterns essential for reconnection.

The transition from convicted offender to free member of the community is especially difficult and complicated because of the value issues that must be resolved for self and others in order to complete the identity transformation. All status-passages are characterized by a concern with personal and social values, since achieving a new identity in any social area requires establishing congruence between the needs and goals of the individual self and the value expectations of others. But in the correctional transitional process the value issue with which the client and his community are engaged is fundamentally moral. The questions to be answered during the correctional transition are these: Is the individual safe to have among us? Can he belong to normal groups without destroying the trust between person and person essential for social life?

Thus the correctional client's task requires him to move from the position of one who has been socially defined as a not-to-be-trusted person to a position in which he is re-established as one who is morally responsible and thus safe for membership in the free community. And since moral values are pervasive in social action, his identity as convicted offender affects all his basic social roles. Grave issues hang on the outcome of each such transitional process, both the destiny of a person as a social being and the formation of community values as they are expressed in control over deviance. The fundamental morality of both the individual and his community are tried and in certain ways modified in the transformation of any convicted offender into a free member of the community.

This analysis of the task leads us to recognize that the primary actors in the correctional client status-passage include not only the offender himself but also his community. The central figure is the offender, the one designated here as the correctional client. But the significant persons in the client's personal community, as well as the community framework of sanctions and resources within which the status-passage endeavor occurs, share responsibility for the ultimate social reconnection, since the offender cannot prove himself morally responsible except through performance in the basic social roles required of every community member. No person can reintegrate in vacuo. Consequently the correctional client's task is one requiring reciprocal changes in himself, in his role partners, and in the community processes affecting them all.

Most normal status-passages provide for a "coach" to assist the individual in moving from one status to another, and this role is often filled by some person who has been through the process himself and who is already warmly related to the central actor. Today in our complex and fragmented society certain status-passage tasks may require the assistance of a professional helper who can guide the individual in managing the personal and social factors involved in identity transformation. Analysis of the correctional client's task suggests that his status-passage is one of those in which most individuals can use some sort of professional facilitation. The value issues at stake are both critical and pervasive, the individual is usually deprived in personal and social resources, and some significant actors may be inaccessible to influence by the client.

Because of the nature of the correctional client's task, the writer views social work as a primary discipline in providing the necessary help. This is not to suggest that all correctional clients need special help—or help provided continuously—or that social work is the only discipline whose assistance is needed to prepare the client for social reconnection. Rather, the social worker is seen as a guide to the process, one who is alert to critical points in the client's experience, who can mobilize needed resources, and who can represent the community's desire for reconnection through an individualized relationship.

Implications for the Agency

This analysis of the client's task in correctional work has major implications for the way the function of the correctional agency is conceptualized. Historically the popular notion of the correctional agency's responsibility—too often naïvely accepted by the professional social worker—is defined as doing something to and for the client that keeps him from bothering the community. As a result correctional agencies now operate with two conflicting social assignments: (1) to protect the community through punishing and segregating the client and (2) to change the client so he becomes an acceptable participant in the community. Agency goals, so formulated, offer opposed models for action and confuse efforts to prescribe how human resources should be organized to accomplish the agency mission, what competence and skills are required for task performance, and what criteria are appropriate for evaluating success and failure. Until there is more clarity about correctional agency goals and the means essential for accomplishing those goals it is nonsense to speak of social work practice in the correctional field.

Accordingly it is proposed that the correctional agency's mission should be defined as establishing for a population of clients the general conditions most favorable for task success. This is a different formulation of agency function from the more usual one of "meeting the client's needs." In contrast this position asserts that the client's needs must be met through normal social processes with his significant others and that the agency is responsible for mobilizing the human relationships involved in social reconnection in a way that encourages the central actors to establish reciprocal need-meeting interaction. This is a probabilistic rather than a deterministic conception of agency function, since in this perspective the agency refuses to take over from the community—whose actions toward the client often determine outcome—total responsibility for success or failure.

The implications of this definition of agency mission for agency organization and for the role of social work in the agency are enormous. Rather than attempting to spell out these implications in abstract propositions, the writer will illustrate what is meant by relating experiences in a prison for young adult offenders.[1]

The Prison Community

Because the project was based in a prison it was first necessary to achieve a realistic idea of what an institution can do to influence the offender's transition toward social reconnection. On his entrance into prison the inmate has been removed from the persons with whom he will associate when he returns to the community, his role partners are in large measure selected for him by the institution, and his whole experience might well seem to him more a suspension of real life than a first step in work on social reconnection. Accordingly the project staff adopted a goal for the new "agency" we were proposing to create that was specific for the phase in the client's transition over which we had control—i.e., to establish the conditions under which the inmate would be encouraged to live today as a morally responsible member of a community. In this way it was hoped to encourage individual inmates (1) to conceive of their recently experienced degradation in social identity as an opportunity to make a new beginning and (2) to establish continuity between their present and future through active preparation for a more successful life on the streets. In short, we wanted these men to be in motion in the right direction,

---

[1] A full report of the prison program discussed is found in Elliot Studt, Sheldon L. Messinger, and Thomas P. Wilson, *C-Unit: Search for Community in Prison* (New York: Russell Sage Foundation, 1968).

equipped with adequate value maps and social skills, when they left the prison's gates.

Pooling Human Resources

Since the goals adopted could only be accomplished through action among the individual inmate and other persons, it was necessary to survey the human resources available for creating real life in prison. Who would be the role partners with whom each inmate would find it necessary to resolve moral issues? To begin with there would be his fellows, 130 at a time, randomly selected, aged 17–30, and housed in C-Unit, one of seven such wings in the institution. Next there would be the staff of twelve to fifteen officials assigned to C-Unit: three master's degree social workers known as counselors, three regular custody officers, two or three secretaries, three researchers, a social worker as administrative supervisor, and the writer as general director of both the research and action programs. In addition there were the many institutional employees who would be related to C-Unit inmates as they participated in the institutional programs for work, education, recreation, and feeding. During the second year there would also be several parole officers from different districts in the state who would be coming periodically to the institution to plan for the parole futures of C-Unit inmates. Finally there would be various representatives of the outside community such as the inmates' family members, volunteers, and students from nearby universities. These persons would constitute the dramatis personae in the first act of the resurrection drama we hoped to initiate. Together they would comprise the human resources available for work on the task of preparing for social reconnection. It was the project's job, as agency, to organize the relationships among these persons in a way that maximized the usefulness of each interaction for task accomplishment.

Creating a Way of Life

Accordingly project staff set out to create a way of life among all the persons affecting the C-Unit inmate's institutional experience that would encourage the establishment of trustworthy relationships and would demonstrate that morally responsible behavior was both necessary and rewarding for members of a community. This meant creating an organization that resembled a community in which responsibility was actually delegated to individuals and groups and in which all activities, no matter how superficially insignificant, would dramatize the fundamental issues of individual needs and group welfare, justice under rules and individual rights, and the encouragement of diversity within a framework of necessary social values. In such a community it was hoped that each inmate would be challenged to work on whatever value problem was involved in his own banishment from and future re-entry into the free community. It was also hoped that most of the inmate's daily activities would become opportunities for him to explore in action a new identity as an acceptable community member.

In the beginning only a few, but nevertheless major, organizational changes were established. Each inmate was assigned the role of member of the C-Unit community, a role he shared with every other inmate in C-Unit and with staff, and an attempt was made to clinch the inmate's membership, for him and for staff, by requiring that he live in C-Unit until he was ready for release from the institution. Staff members were freed from their isolating memberships in hierarchical subdivisions within the institution—custody, counselors, secretaries, researchers—and established as members of a staff work group under a single administration. The staff was made responsible as a group for the agency's impact on the total C-Unit population. Finally, these various kinds of community members were set to work at solving the real problems of their daily lives together.

The community structure and its program of activities emerged with staff help from the common engagement with tasks that were meaningful to both staff and inmates. These tasks and problems were basically those concerned with the day-to-day life of the community. It did not really matter whether the problem at hand was noise in the television room, disruption caused by poor communication among staff members, rising tension during a holiday period, or the handling of a schizophrenic inmate who was hallucinating. Each identified problem concerned inmates as well as staff and both had a stake in problem resolution and a contribution to make. As modes for analyzing problems and for mobilizing the appropriate problem-solving skills were tried out, community patterns for work were established and community values became evident in shared norms.

No one knew ahead of time that community would first emerge as a matter of pride among the C-Unit inmates in their unpremeditated but uniform refusal to participate in an institutional riot and in their overriding concern for the safety of each C-Unit inmate during the riot period, or that by the end of the eighth month a major project would be a C-Unit Inmate Welfare Fund from which needy inmates could draw money to purchase the grooming aids and small luxuries available at the canteen, or that the contribution of money from inmates would eventuate in a fund to be used for "the good of the whole," making possible a unit library as well as other amenities. Such activities—the newspaper, the football team, the monthly dinners that include C-Unit inmates and staff together with other officials from the larger institutional staff, the holiday open houses with visitors from the community, the many kinds of interest groups ranging in focus from concern with race relationships or the problems of job-seeking to learning about art or music—might on the surface seem to have been time-filling pursuits similar to what people do anywhere in the use of leisure time. Similarity between activities in prison and life on the outside was perceived as good in itself, but the staff also valued the fact that such activities provided opportunities for these social outcasts to act in their own behalf while learning to resolve such issues as potential conflict between subgroup needs and community welfare or between individual interests and the need for social control over the means by which individuals pursue their own goals.

Equally important was what the staff learned through the spontaneous individual and group developments that appeared as soon as the agency became in fact a process for organizing human resources in a way that established conditions favorable to work on the client's tasks. It was first learned that the kind of work group the staff created for itself out of its own relationships determined in large measure the quality of problem-solving in the official program where staff and inmates worked together and the quality of the relationships the inmates established among themselves. All data, both positive and negative, showed clearly that when staff were in conflict, fragmented, and evasive with each other, "shuck" and "front" took over in the relations between staff and inmates and conflict groups appeared among the inmates.[2] It was equally evident that when the staff were task focused, openly sharing information, undefensively analyzing problems, and contributing without regard to hierarchical differences, similar problem-solving processes appeared in action among the inmates.

Staff also learned that it was not necessary to try to break the inmate system in order to influence inmate norms in support of staff values. A survey of inmate systems in the institution at the end of C-Unit's first year supported observational data in suggesting that C-Unit had a stronger inmate system than did other units. However, the C-Unit system was unique in the institution because its norms supported its members in working with staff for individual and group welfare. The strategy for influencing the inmate system was a simple one. Staff legitimated inmate interests, usually served only by sub rosa inmate activities, by making these the concern of staff as well as of inmates, and the agency was designed as a set of means by which the inmates with the help of the staff, could pursue their legitimate interests. Overall, the C-Unit experience proved abundantly that prison inmates are not necessarily antistaff and that, given the chance, they became the active members of the agency work force it was anticipated they would be.

This pooling of human resources for flexible use made possible the spontaneous development of quite different kinds of treatment strategies in response to the different needs and capacities of different kinds of inmates. These strategies used all the ongoing relationships in the life of the individual inmate—with counselors, custodians, teachers, parole officer, and fellow inmates—to reinforce and complement the contributions of each to preparation for social reconnection. Each such team was led by the inmate's

---

[2] "Shuck" and "front" are terms inmates use to refer to the act of presenting oneself falsely to staff as concerned with social values and rehabilitation in order to get special favors and recommendations for early release.

counselor. In action these teams were quite different from those formed when independent experts, each representing a different discipline, gather for occasional case conferences and divide responsibility among themselves. The C-Unit treatment team evoked an aware, purposive, and pervasive action system with the individual inmate as the central figure, permitting leadership roles to shift as needs varied, as well as in-and-out participation by various persons as some became more and others less salient in the inmate's experience. Such an action system could operate in response to momentary contingencies outside the professional purview because each actor was in some way aware of the goals and governing values, and it could continue to be effective without formal convening of the persons involved. In many cases this group of significant persons, rather than a single "treater," became the socializing "personal community" that made daily life in prison real life and therefore a preparation for the individual inmate's return to the free community.

For the professional social workers on the staff the C-Unit experience meant an expanded image of social work, especially for those caseworkers who entered the experience fearing they might lose their professional skills through doing many things formerly not perceived as part of the method in which they had been trained. Of special importance for such persons was the value added when they assumed a responsible share in planning how the agency would establish the conditions on which their work and that of the inmates depended. The counselors, together with the rest of the staff work group, became the agency in action, and what they had made they could change whenever new perceptions of the task or new needs indicated that change should be made. Furthermore, the community setting greatly facilitated casework diagnosis, helping to distinguish disruptive behaviors that were symptoms of personality disturbance from those that were situationally caused. And the expanded range of ways to intervene in a problem enriched the content of action to be examined in casework interviews, heightened the effectiveness of any one treatment method through reinforcement by other means of influence carrying the same message, and encouraged economy of effort through selectivity in the choice of approaches to specific problems.

Deterioration of the Community

Staff also learned negatively through failure. During the second year the C-Unit community deteriorated. Staff interests and those of inmates were increasingly perceived as opposed; subgroups among staff members as well as among inmates competed with each other for power and privileges, sometimes with great bitterness, and treatment once again became what was done in private between the counselor and an individual inmate, a process essentially in conflict with the pervasive routine activities required by institutional management.

Three major causes were identified for this disintegration of what had been co-ordinated work by many on a common task: (1) C-Unit was required to maintain in its ongoing structure the methods used by the larger institution for the control of undesirable behavior, e.g., the rules defining deviance, the processes for determining which acts were deviant, the punishments used, and the formal rewards for conformity. By the end of the first year it became increasingly evident that the means used for the control of behavior are critical for the treatment of deviants and that no real community can exist unless the principles that govern its response to deviant behavior are the same as those governing its welfare activities. (2) Gradually responsibility was removed from the staff work group and bureaucratic, hierarchical authority patterns were reinstituted by new management in the C-Unit community. (3) The ultimate cause of dissolution lay in the increasingly evident divergence between the principles of action used by the larger institution's authorities and the problem-solving principles on which the C-Unit community was established. The opposed patterns characteristic of the larger agency and of the small demonstration agency within it could not be reconciled by efforts from the subordinate unit alone. Eventually C-Unit re-established within itself the divisive management practices of the total institution rather than becoming the instrument for change it was designed to be.

It should not be assumed, however, that nothing of value occurred because the C-Unit experiment failed to stabilize the problem-solving culture of its first year. Rather, we learned that it is important to live with an agency through an apparent short-run failure in a way that helps administrators learn what is necessary in the long run to support their announced goals for change and increased effectiveness. Today the institution in which C-Unit is housed has been reorganized throughout, using many concepts developed in the C-Unit community. The unit approach to grouping staff and inmates has been picked up by other institutions in the state to good advantage. And the state Department of Corrections is now supporting a thorough study of parole services in preparation for a similar demonstration program in parole, with considerably more sophistication about the commitments and costs required to make such an endeavor successful. Thus the C-Unit community may be termed a qualified success, with much to teach us about the complex factors involved in changing old bureaucracies so they can support new services and about the time it takes to translate therapeutic ideas into stabilized organizational action.

Relevance for the Parole Process

As C-Unit inmates left the institution it became increasingly evident that the correctional client's adaptive task on re-entry into the community was in certain ways even more difficult than that he faced on admission to the institution and that clients on parole needed the same kind of agency facilitation as we attempted to provide in the institution. Accordingly, during the years since the C-Unit project, some of those associated with the C-Unit project have been examining the parole process to see if what was learned might have relevance for organizing the persons who help to determine parole outcome. So far our studies have identified certain dimensions of the parolee's task that call for adaptations in the C-Unit model for parole agency design, although the basic principles seem as appropriate for social work in the field service as in the institution.

In C-Unit when we wanted to change an institutional program for a process for "doing something to people" into a set of conditions supporting the work of clients, we found it necessary to make three kinds of structural changes: (1) we made the client an active member of the agency, (2) we delegated responsibility for designing the agency-in-action to a staff work group, and (3) we involved the client's significant role partners in appropriate task-related agency roles. As we changed the relationships among the persons who were important to task outcomes, we found that the "shape" and function of the agency changed. It was no longer the traditional bureaucratic, limiting "frame" for the activities of the caseworker. Rather it was better described as a flow of mutually reinforcing human activities, each of which could be used flexibly as a resource. The agency itself became a treatment tool, communicating to the inmates the moral values of the "good society" and thus helping to prepare prison inmates for futures in the free community.

The adaptations of the C-Unit model required by conditions in the field arise directly from the nature of the correctional client's task once he is released to the open community. Here he is involved in actual social reconnection rather than in preparation. His work on the task occurs in those relationships that will hopefully become his permanent personal community—in his home, his work, his activities as a consumer, and his use of leisure time—rather than in daily interchange with agency officials. This fact has many implications for agency structure in the field service.

In parole the significant persons affecting the task outcome are widely dispersed and often they are not even aware of others in the task-related network. These significant others tend to hold conflicting goals and expectations for the parolee and may act in ways that disrupt what others are trying to accomplish. At the same time the client moves alone among these relationships as a stigmatized person surrounded by free people. In most normal roles his position is weak, although in each he is expected to behave as though he were both independent and adequate; in contrast, his role with the agency emphasizes his dependent and restricted membership in the community. The formal agency responsible for guiding the client in his adaptive efforts influences the social reconnection process primarily through a caseworker—the parole agent—who works in isolation from his colleagues while performing many agency functions for each client in his dispersed case load. Furthermore, wherever the parole agent moves in his client's life he makes explicit the parolee's degraded status simply by his official presence even when his intention is to help. In addition the agency represents the power of the state to return the parolee to prison as well as the intention of the community to help, thus introducing conflicts for both the parolee and the agent into the process of gathering the information needed to facilitate social reconnection.[3]

Thus each parolee tends to spend his life interacting with persons who are psychologically and socially distant from each other, all unaware that their combined actions will determine the success or failure of social reconnection efforts. Such a system of action is normally characterized by interrupted communications, distorted information, ambiguous or conflicting expectations, and unilateral decision-making. Our studies already reveal that most parolees' lives are, in fact, severely fragmented and subject to unanticipated crises that can be widely disruptive throughout the tenuous new relationships each is attempting to establish. Accordingly, organizing the parole agency to support social reconnection requires finding some way to co-ordinate the activities of the many individuals who are contributing to parole outcomes. At this stage of our study we are better able to document the problems to be anticipated in such an attempt than to prescribe the shape of a more effective parole agency. However, we do have some educated guesses about the patterns for work that should characterize a future "C-Unit in paroles."

Staff Work Group

The obvious first step would be to do something about the current fragmentation among the employees of the official agency, since these persons are most easily affected by administrative direction, and the staff work group responsible for an identifiable population of parole clients suggests itself as the most appropriate

---

[3] For greater detail concerning these problems *see* Elliot Studt, *The Reentry of the Offender into the Community,* No. 9002 (Washington, D.C.: Office of Juvenile Delinquency and Youth Development, U.S. Department of Health, Education & Welfare, 1967).

means for starting co-ordinated work. In the agency studied, such a unit of operations would be the supervisory unit with its supervisor, six or seven agents, one or more secretaries, and possibly a psychiatric consultant, who together share responsibility for 250–400 parolees living in a given geographic area. Organization of these persons as a work group would encourage them to pool information about the needs evidenced in their shared case load and to deploy their combined official resources in response to these needs. Of major importance, such an arrangement would encourage the development of a colleague-enforced system of values to guide the individual agent's exercise of discretion as he represents the agency in decision-making with parolees and other task-related persons.

The Parolee As Co-worker

A first assignment to such a staff work group would be to discover means to engage the parolees as active co-workers on the task of social reconnection. A major finding of our exploratory studies is that the dependent, supervised role currently established for the parolee in relationship with the official agency is so incongruent with the expectations of his "normal" life roles that it frequently introduces additional strains into an already difficult undertaking. Since the parolee has limited means for influencing what the agent does about his life, most parolees are evasive about sharing information and hesitant to ask for help even when faced with complications they cannot manage on their own. Finding some means by which parolees can act vigorously on their own behalf with the agency seems necessary if they are to behave as free men as they go about their normal social duties.

An obvious difficulty in the parolee's role with the agency, as it is now defined, is the negative nature of the rules administered by the agent and the added fact that rule ambiguity gives each agent wide latitude for making idiosyncratic decisions about the personal life of each parolee. No parolee is encouraged to involve his agent in thoughtful consideration of pros and cons when he knows that an unexplained "no" on the part of the agent can deny him permission to drive, to buy a car, to move across county lines, to change his job, or to take any one of a number of actions that seem necessary if he is to get about his business of living a normal life in the community. The rules of parole are not easy to change; legislative enactments, the parole board, and the Department of Corrections all share responsibility for maintaining the "custody in the community" concept of parolees that is embodied in the list of parole rules. But as they now stand, these conditions of parole define the parolee as helpless to make any major and many minor decisions on his own, and they must be either modified or reinterpreted if the parolee is to see himself in any sense as a co-worker with parole officials.

Once the parole role is designed so that agents and parolees can conceive of themselves as co-workers, it will be necessary to plan activities through which the parolees can contribute their knowledge of problems and their resources to the common task. It is not easy to describe just what activities would establish the parolees in a given client population as contributing members of the agency's working force without some knowledge of the concrete problems met by a specific set of parolees. But from what we have learned by following a panel of parolees from prerelease through the first year of parole, we can sketch a number of functions that almost any case load of parolees could usefully perform in influencing the way the agency seeks to support social reconnection.

First, it is clear that parolees should be more actively involved in identifying and specifying commonly experienced problems, including those caused by agency policies and practices. I could see in almost any parole case load a number of parole groups, brought together not for some vague counseling or therapeutic goal, but because the members of each were commonly concerned with core problems such as obtaining employment, budgeting and purchasing, how to fill leisure time, problems encountered with welfare agencies and the police, or the ambiguities inherent in parole rules. Such groups can easily be turned into resources not only for understanding the nature of the problems but also for inventing solutions and mobilizing resources in the parolees' own lives.

Such group activity is not useful or necessary for all parolees nor is it seen as a continuing form of participation for many, although all would benefit by having their role in the agency changed from that of subject to co-worker. In the institution, group activity among inmates was an essential dimension of institutional living; the C-Unit plan simply made use of the facts of daily life. But in the community there are some parolees whose normal group experiences are adequate for personal problem-solving and for whom enforced association with other parolees would serve no useful function. For the large number of parolees, however, legitimate and mutually useful activities with others who share the same status would provide much-needed support during the early months on parole and would offer mechanisms through which even such disadvantaged persons might gain the enhancement of self-worth that comes from helping others. As we learned in the C-Unit experience, one cannot anticipate the specific patterns of work that might emerge as parolees are offered the opportunity to use agency membership for work at shared problems. But the writer has heard enough parolees talk about isolation, loneliness, lack of access to social resources, discomfort in normal groups, and feelings of indignity, impotence, and confusion in relation to the agency to feel sure that pooling agency and parolee resources for joint work on such problems could help turn the parole agency from a handicapping factor in the lives of many parolees into a launching pad toward social reconnection.

Significant Others

Perhaps the agency's involvement with the parolee's significant others is the most problematical area for consideration by the staff work group and the parolee members of the agency. It is unfortunately a fact that many persons and agencies in the nonparolee community do not really want to readmit the parolees to normal membership and tend to look on the agency, not as a support for their own efforts to assist in social reconnection, but as an official means for keeping the parolee from bothering them. In addition, as we have already noted, whenever the parole agency moves into a parolee's life officially there is the danger of spreading stigma, severely diminishing both the parolee's control over the spread of information about himself and his capacity to build a new life for himself.

Even in this sensitive area, however, work by agents and parolees together has proved it is possible to reduce the handicaps of public apathy, disrespect, and disconnection in the lives of certain groups of parolees. One program for addicted parolees has used a parolee group formed to work on the development of educational resources seeking to modify the restrictive policies of a number of schools; another group in the same program has undertaken to provide a public service through offering speakers on the problems of drug addiction to various community groups and in this way has opened up wider resources for the employment of addicts while increasing public understanding of parolees and their potentialities. Ultimately it may be necessary to form multiservice agencies to serve many kinds of deviants in order to reduce the stigma against any one group that follows official intervention whenever an agency represents a special deviant group. Although we are not yet at that stage in parole, it is necessary to find immediate means for co-ordinating the work of others in the community for the positive goal of keeping parolees in the community, rather than as so often happens waiting for the breakdown in social relationships that results in a community demand that a specific parolee be returned to prison.

Certainly we do need to re-examine our usual assumption that the client is the only individual in the social reconnection task who needs to change and to consider with great care the way the client's various official and personal role partners contribute to the success or failure of social reconnection and how they can be helped to become positive forces in the achievement of the task they share with the client. And we need to give much more attention to helping the community create the marginal roles through which identified deviants can satisfy both their own identity needs and the community's need for a certain level of conformity.

The Process of Change

All social workers are concerned in one way or another with the development of new or improved services for deviants. The

C-Unit experience has taught that at least two perspectives are crucial for success in planned change, especially when it envisions adjustments in basic organizational dimensions such as the role of the client in the agency, relationships among staff members, and the way the agency functions toward the client's various role partners.

1. A period of intensive study of the agency processes to be changed seems to be essential if one is to avoid unanticipated and undesirable consequences as a result of the change. During such a preliminary study one can discover the connections among organizational units on which the functioning of each depends. Identifying what actually happens in current operations allows one to be selective in proposing those among all possible changes that are most economical and that give most promise of accomplishing the stated goals. It also permits one to take into account the way organizational dimensions that cannot be changed at the beginning can be expected to affect the proposed new services. The process of study itself helps administrators and others understand the reasons for change and to participate in the choices among alternative means for achieving ends. In addition preliminary study establishes baselines against which the new program can be evaluated. In fact, in our parole study we are finding that the study process itself is the beginning of change action, both providing the information needed for sound program design and preparing personnel at many levels for the new approach in the making of which they will have had a part.

2. In designing any agency as a process for establishing favorable conditions for client work, experience in C-Unit suggests it is critically important to remember that one thing leads to another. Change in one aspect of an agency's organization requires reciprocal changes in all other relevant role relationships or the initial change goes sour, resulting in undesirable consequences for the clients. If one restores client dignity by making him a responsible member of the agency work force, then one must consider changes in the way the official members of the agency relate not only to him but to each other. These changes in turn must be supported by reciprocal changes in upper administration and in the way the agency relates to other parts of the community. Unless such change

problems are anticipated and dealt with as professionally as one deals with the relationship between the social worker and his client, *that* relationship itself will remain, in operation, simply a cover-up process for applying community pressures to isolate and control the deviant client.

Social reconnection of deviants, the facilitation of which is a primary social work function, is not accomplished by the caseworker and his individual client working together in isolation. This fact has implications for social work theories of intervention and for the methods of intervention the profession develops and teaches. Even more urgently, as we move into bold new service designs we need to pay attention to the nature of the client's task when the goal is the return of the deviant person to the free community, and to what this means for organizing the work of the many different persons who make a difference for the accomplishment of the task. Increasingly social scientists are pointing out that bureaucracy is a poor model for any agency whose function is concerned with the present and future welfare of individuals. Social work, of all the helping professions, should be especially concerned with exploring and developing organizational models that can be effective in releasing human creativity, encouraging the development of common value systems, promoting flexibility of response, and establishing viable connections between alienated people and the social matrices within which they must find their ongoing social and personal satisfactions. In the process of learning to relate staff members and others in new patterns we must also focus more carefully on the steps involved in planned organizational change and on the skills required to mobilize all available human resources for the accomplishment of client tasks.

Themes of leadership

Jerome Cohen

The aim of the Leadership Training Program of the National Association of Social Workers has been the identification and further development of social work leadership in the mental health field. The purpose of this paper is, through assuming an integrative task, to illuminate those qualities revealed by the program's attempt to define the nature of that illusive activity called leadership.

The accretion of experience reaffirms an earlier recognition that healthy progress and development do not call for the obliteration of past skill and knowledge. One need not destroy in healthy development that which has been a part of one's prior identity. The ability to respecify and restructure professional knowledge and role is at least as important as the mastery of additional knowledge and skills related to the new tasks. Successful mastery of this developmental task requires the ability to synthesize both new knowledge and personal attributes with previous experiences and behavior. Changes in professional direction need not be accompanied by an abrupt and massive revolutionary trend. Destruction and dissolution of old themes and regimes may be necessary on occasion, but this is not a viable means of normal progression in any developmental process, whether individual or institutional.

It is important also to emphasize that energies must be related to the broad values and purposes of social work in order to avoid the manipulation of individuals and systems for personal ends. We ought not to be concerned with the lexicographer's definition of leadership as "the development of conditions which entitle one to precedence over his associates." We ought to be more organized toward the alternate definition of "one who molds individuals into a team for the successful resolution of problems." This is especially urgent when the issue of power is dealt with. As Wax wrote: "The professional is first and foremost accountable to his own sense of professional identity and integrity. His education provides the framework and knowledge and values within which other influences must operate." [1]

Characteristics and Qualities of Leadership

The movement from latent or potential to manifest leadership roles frequently requires a new perspective on the investment of time. Assuming leadership in any field requires a greater commitment of time and energy. There is no way to influence the structure of action without a willingness to invest heavily in activities that affect one's ability to influence others. This demands continual involvement in knowledge-building activities, engagement in formal and informal relationships with those whose alliance is critical to one's cause, and acceptance of the depletion of energy attendant on the variety of stress factors inherent in leadership positions. The intention here is not to depress and discourage those who seek leadership roles but rather to be realistic about the requisites of such a role. For those who are of a mind and spirit to make the investment there are many rewards.

Leadership also requires the ability to accept *measured risks—* "measured" because leadership does not demand blind, aggressive

---

[1] John Wax, "Social Process and Social Work Accountability in the Mental Hospital," *International Journal of Social Psychiatry,* Vol. 13, No. 4 (1967), pp. 297–300.

action with threats inherent in every engagement. Rather, it requires the ability to evaluate the conditions that prevail in relation
to a specific desired end. Attention will be given later to issues
of influence, power, and knowledge of systems that enable one to
measure the potential for change. It is nevertheless true that the
"buck" stops upon the assumption of leadership. There is no way
of avoiding the fact that the moment of truth comes when one can
no longer say, "Let George do it." When the individual has measured the situation as well as he possibly can and believes that the
issues and stakes are high enough for him to take a stand, it is he,
as a leader, who must be willing to risk himself to achieve the
goal. In leadership roles there is little opportunity to join those
who in their professional alienation continue to cry, "*They* won't
let us do it." It is an attitude that is reflected rather than a specific behavior. There are few instances in which professionals are
forced to place themselves in jeopardy to achieve the objectives
they value, but there are many instances in which this possibility
must be recognized as a potential consequence.

However, new risks also bring about new opportunity: the
opportunity to use skills and knowledge in the most creative way
possible, the opportunity to participate in deciding on the direction in which institutional and professional energies are to be used,
and—most critical—the opportunity to implement those programs
and plans that are viewed as important to the well-being of the
populations served. The new role enables one to become a part
of new reference groups within the institution and the larger community that supports it. One begins to associate with planning
bodies related to service delivery. One finds oneself with new alliances and new experiences that emerge out of the development of
those alliances, with the potential for developing new resources to
carry out the ideas one has helped create, and, it is hoped, with a
mastery of new knowledge and sense of competence.

Leadership, then, is not a matter of gambling. It requires the
use of knowledge to keep the element of risk at the lowest level
possible. It is necessary to know when to use a power base for
change in a system and when not to lose one's cool with a pre-
mature response. In the long run the difference between being in

charge of a unit and being a leader in that unit hinges on the capacity to evaluate correctly opportunity and, understanding the
geography of a situation, to take advantage of it to move toward
goals.

Other attributes of leadership closely resemble characteristics of
the generally mature or competent individual. For example, a
critical faculty is the ability to *give* comfortably as well as to
receive comfortably, to be able to trust in others as well as to
enable others to trust you, to have the capacity to seek recognition
for others and to ascribe to others the advantages and recognition
that you may have achieved—in other words, to risk yourself for
a collectivity and then pass on to the collectivity that which you
have been able to achieve. As promises are kept and recognition
and concern for others voiced and acted on, one will find a growing
account in the institutional bank of influence.

Knowledge Base for Leadership

Of the many knowledge themes presented in the Leadership
Training Program, Beck's injunction to focus on a problem orientation is one of the most critical to social work's expanding practice.[2] It is the key to extending awareness from individual adaptation to the needs of specific populations while still maintaining the
depth of understanding required of professional intervention. Once
services are organized around a target population characterized by
a specific kind of problem behavior, the door has been opened to
a variety of interventions previously beyond the scope of social
work's perceptions and efforts. As attention is given to an entire
population rather than only to those individuals who are screened
through intake devices of a specific organization, new parameters
of the problem emerge that were previously hidden or avoided.
Not only do the problems become more manifest, but new resources
are uncovered that were not considered part of the previous set of
interventive actions. Institutions, both formal and informal—

---

[2] Bertram M. Beck, "A Social Work Approach to a Mental Health Objective,"
this volume, pp. 61–71.

storefront churches, ward politicians, gangs, extended kinship net-
works, and so on—are found within the population at risk as
well as potential nonprofessional resources to help reach organizational goals.

Such perspectives directly affect the nature of social work strategies. It now becomes necessary to be concerned with the interre-
lationship of the clinic or institutional population, the community
from which this limited and selected population derives, and the
broad social policy and program that affect the structure of action
in that community. Movement is then from client to the broader
population from which the client comes and finally to the broad
community action system—political, social, and economic—that
affects the behavior of its members; in this way social work's efforts
are tied to the social issues of our time.

One of the emphases in the Leadership Training Program has
been the provision of a beginning perspective on the organizational
knowledge that must be developed to carry out the new tasks of this
changing practice. If we react only with computer phobias when
a systems approach to mental health problems is introduced, then
we miss an opportunity to enrich our perspectives of concrete system interrelationships that affect, in a specific way, the work done
in individual settings. The content of a basic data pool, the in-depth
knowledge of personal and institutional resources, and the means
by which individuals can be located who are in need but whose
disability is manifested in ways that do not bring them to an
agency's attention—in these areas skill and sophistication must
be developed to achieve stated goals.

Studt carried the message of this insight into the direct practice
elements of the social worker's role.[3] She set out the tasks of the
social work practitioner in a manner not really unfamiliar, that of
facilitating the successful resolution of the client's task—in this
case, becoming reconnected socially to the nondeviant sector of
the community. Studt identified the adaptive tasks necessary to
carry out that goal and in so doing was able once more to see the
impact on behavior of the many interrelated systems affecting the

---

[3] Elliot Studt, "Deviant Roles and Social Reconnection," this volume, pp.
72–92.

life of her clients. She discarded the assumption that the client's problem was *inevitably* a condition located only within himself and that therefore resolution of his problem involved changing in some way the nature of his self-system. She has respecified the central component of the social work perspective: the reality of a psychosocial explanation of behavior and the intervention necessary to change that behavior. The social space and the various institutional systems become the arena of action for the successful resolution of adaptive tasks in the process of becoming reconnected to the community. More and more this is seen to be relevant to those who have been defined as mentally ill. Studt's perspective is no less true for the status passage from hospital to community than it is from prison to community. The theory she presented is helpful because it offers a clear basis for actions toward goals that can be defined and evaluated.

The direction of Litwak's work, whether this aspect of his linkage theory is validated or requires change, represents still another aspect of knowledge without which leadership is impotent: the specificity between goals and actions exemplified in his work.[4] Once a perspective such as this has been mastered it can be used at a level of intervention known in only a few social and psychological theories. If one is to be effective then one must be prepared to offer one's colleagues and institutions specific goal-related prescriptions for action capable of evaluation. This kind of risk can be avoided only at the peril of one's professional development and the relinquishment of the leadership role.

It is also necessary to understand the nature of organizations and the specific type of organization that can most effectively serve a particular purpose. It is not likely that we shall return to the romantic joys of Redfield's "folk society" in which primary groups alone suffice to meet the needs of the population.[5] Short of massive destruction on this planet, which in order to maintain a measure of sanity we must assume will not occur, it will be necessary

---

[4] Eugene Litwak, "Toward a Balance Theory of Grass-Roots Community Organization," this volume, pp. 22–60.
[5] Robert Redfield, *The Little Community: Peasant Society and Culture* (Chicago: University of Chicago Press, 1960).

to deal with increasing numbers and types of organizations. Witness the poverty areas, which were previously characterized mainly by primary group organizations and are now moving toward the more formal type of organizations that may make it possible for them to achieve new goals.

As Litwak points out, the rational bureaucracy is characterized by formal and clearly defined patterns of activity in which ideally every series of actions is functionally related to the purpose of the organization.[6] Toward this end people are selected and promoted on the basis of their ability and knowledge alone, thus maximizing the knowledge available to the organization. Such organizations demand specialization and the use of highly developed skill and knowledge characterized by a generalized systematic practice. Specific organizational goals are the basis for decision-making and there is an a priori definition of duties and privileges that tends to avoid the introduction of personal goals. The rules are universalistic and common decision-making policies prevail for all segments of the organization. This means that written rules are the order of the day and are not to be departed from except under specific conditions. When such conditions prevail there is a hierarchical ladder of authority to which all parts of the organization are subjected.

The primary group, on the other hand, stresses strong positive affect rather than impersonal relations. One does things for others because one cares for them regardless of their abilities, and preservation of close ties is seen as an end in itself. The continuity of the group is a major goal overshadowing functional tasks outside it. Rather than a stress on specialization, diffuse relations are found in which duties and obligations may be transferred from one person to another. The stress is on face-to-face contact rather than written memorandums. Such groups must therefore remain small throughout their history. Using this knowledge, Litwak offers a contribution to the assignment of duties to a wide range of social work practitioners. He suggests that a primary group member or nonprofessional may be more appropriate for a task when (1) that task is simple enough for a nonexpert to accomplish it (the

---

[6] *Op. cit.*

important point is that when both *can* do it the nonprofessional *ought* to do it), (2) there is no body of knowledge, so experts cannot be trained, and, perhaps most important, (3) the situation is so complex or unexpected that expert knowledge cannot be brought to bear in time. In this last classification may be found many of the serious pathologies and problems with which social workers deal. At a time when the use of many different levels of personnel is becoming necessary as well as desirable, a method of determining the appropriate time and circumstance when each should be used is of major importance.

Administrative-Professional Conflict

Another aspect of bureaucratic organization requires some mention because of its direct impact on the structure of professional action. Etzioni in his writings on modern organizations has pointed out the structural dilemma and strain imposed by the conflicting perspectives of administrative and professional authority.[7] Administration frequently, if not always, assumes an ultimate power hierarchy. There is a ranking of decision-making apparatus such that the higher the administrative rank, the more prerogatives one has on ultimate control and co-ordination of other organizational members' activities. This control and co-ordination can, of course, be transferred in formal ways to other persons, but the basic principle of organization as a rational and co-ordinated system requires this formal arrangement. Professional creativity and knowledge are another matter altogether. These attributes cannot be transferred at will from one to another through the medium of a written memorandum. The creation of autonomy necessary for professionals to make decisions based on knowledge and competence has long been a critical problem within the social work profession as well as within other types of organizations using professional personnel. Etzioni suggests:

> The ultimate justification for a professional act is that it is, to the best of the professional's knowledge, the right act. He might

---

[7] Amitai Etzioni, *Modern Organizations* (Englewood Cliffs, N.J.: Prentice-Hall, 1964).

consult his colleagues before he acts, but the decision is his. If he errs, he still will be defended by his peers. The ultimate justification of an administrative act, however, is that it is in line with the organization's rules and regulations, and that it has been approved—directly or by implication—by a superior rank.[8]

How to bring social work's knowledge and viewpoint to changes needed in organizational direction, given the hierarchical position the profession occupies in the mental health system, is a factor that cannot be ignored. But the task of leadership not only requires a consideration of one's relationship to those above one in the hierarchy of administration, it also requires attention to the way in which one relates to those lower in the hierarchical administrative order. Leaders in mental health organizations share both an administrative and professional role. Organizational demands of the administrative function are often those of evaluation and control. This aspect of agency structure allows for the degrees of responsibility necessary in a system of accountability. Yet the same person is in another sense also called on to create an environment in which professional practitioner autonomy can be expanded and greater opportunity for decision-making and self-direction provided. Such dilemmas and role conflict need to be understood. One of the responsibilities of leadership personnel is to find new forms of organizational behavior that will allow for a more productive relationship between the practicing professional and the administrative forces within the organization.

Some leaders in social work have begun to point the way in their contributions to the literature on supervision. Those who have written as well as demonstrated in their own organizations that some modification is possible, such as John Wax and Ruth Fizdale, begin with a firm and honest belief in the wisdom of maximizing the autonomy and responsibility of practitioners.[9] They

---

[8] *Ibid.,* p. 77.

[9] *See,* for example, John Wax, "Time-Limited Supervision," *Social Work,* Vol. 8, No. 3 (July 1963), pp. 37–43; Ruth Fizdale, "Peer Group Supervision," *Social Casework,* Vol. 39, No. 8 (October 1958), pp. 443–450.

respect the authority of ideas rather than solely the ascribed authority of administrative position with a conviction that allows them to permit authority to flow from competence. But they recognize that such values and beliefs require of them a further responsibility to supply the resources for practitioners to reach the highest level of competence of which they are capable. They are engaged in constant search for the development of resources to increase the competence and thereby the reputation and impact of the practitioner. In the process they have created new potentials for practitioner participation in policy-making and have provided a growing sense of trust among the staff that limits the necessity to engage in constant control functions.

Development of Relevant Power

There is also, however, the necessity for concern with the issues of power relevant to bringing about change in the organizations and communities of one's everyday work. The work of Wax comes to mind once more. He has been the most articulate leader in the profession concerning the ingredients of leadership itself and the necessary knowledge base as well as values to, as he puts it, "make things happen." A few of the important dimensions of his prescriptions for the development of relevant power follow.[10]

Power is available in both formal and informal ways. We have talked about the power inherent in the administrative line functioning of rational bureaucratic organizations. It is well to remember that it also resides in such informal situations as the "gatekeeper" function. To be a friend of the gatekeeper in a treatment organization is often to have access to one of the most powerful allies one can have. To *be* the gatekeeper is to wield power of considerable magnitude. Social work has often held this responsibility without recognizing its potential meaning. For example, social workers are most frequently used as intake personnel in treatment organizations. Much has been written about the technical issues related to

---

[10] *See* John Wax, "Relevant Power." Unpublished paper presented at the NASW Leadership Training Program, Chicago, Ill., April 1968.

the intake function but not a single article in the social work literature describes the way in which such a function can shape an entire institution's program and directions. In a study of social mobility and public housing in which the writer participated some years ago, it was discovered that the character of a city's public housing program was determined in a major way by a clerk who made the first decision as to who was to be considered for residence in any of the quite different public housing projects of that community.[11] This is influence worth thinking about. This is the kind of potential for making things happen that must not be overlooked.

Wax also reminds us that the structure of power is not fixed in a "monolithic system of decision-making which controls the entire community or institutions." This is especially true in professional organizations. There is always some degree of departure from the ideal of a bureaucratic organization with a straight line of hierarchical control in decision-making. In any event, influencing the decision-making process can often be achieved by developing alliances that impel decision-makers to consider seriously the consequences of their action. In reality decisions are made at all levels of an organization and by many different groups within it. It is not only wise but necessary to make alliances with as many individuals and groups as possible so that support may be found for the influence one would like to bring to bear on the directions of the organization's behavior.

Conclusion

If all this sounds enervating, it is. The investment of such energies needs to be harnessed for social rather than personal ends. Herein lies the fear and aversion many social workers have felt in regard to the concept of power and the seeking of influence. This does not mean that they have not often engaged in such activities but rather that it was not recognized in polite professional company.

---

[11] Irwin Deutscher, "The Gatekeeper in Public Housing," in Deutscher and Elizabeth Thompson, eds., *Among the People* (New York: Basic Books, 1968), pp. 38–53.

The fear that power might be used for personal rather than social ends does, of course, recognize a real danger. All the more important for social workers to be aware of the value base on which we operate. We have previously looked to institutional controls to assure that the directions of our practice would be related to the value system espoused. In the field of mental health institutions have frequently not only failed to assure such directions but have often developed systems that have opposite consequences from those espoused. When cure was valued, illness has been encouraged. It is time to accept the personal responsibility inherent in leadership in an effort to return to a more congruent relationship between value and function.

Above all the leader is a realist. He must be aware not only of the desirable but also of the possible. An awareness of the degrees of freedom in a situation must when necessary be evaluated as carefully as the potential for change.

The most difficult task of all is the application of general knowledge to the specific situation within which one has to operate. How to particularize the theories and principles discussed here for one's own situation is the hardest job of all. We speak of a strategy with a capital "S" and you must find the strategy with a small "s." We speak of populations with a capital "P" and you must find the answers for a population with a small "p." You cannot use canned knowledge any more effectively than research investigators can use canned programs on a computer and still be effective. The knowledge needs to be suited to specific circumstances. This requires the ability to modify and reconceptualize the nature of the action so that it can be carried out under the conditions that actually prevail "where it's at" for you in your organization and in your community.

6/70–1½ M–P&K